D1480428

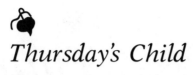

Thursday's Child

Thursday's

Child

VICTORIA POOLE

Little, Brown and Company — Boston–Toronto

COPYRIGHT © 1980 BY VICTORIA SIMES POOLE

ALL RIGHTS RESERVED. NO PART OF THIS BOOK MAY BE REPRODUCED IN ANY FORM OR BY ANY ELECTRONIC OR MECHANICAL MEANS INCLUDING INFORMATION STORAGE AND RETRIEVAL SYSTEMS WITHOUT PERMISSION IN WRITING FROM THE PUBLISHER, EXCEPT BY A REVIEWER WHO MAY QUOTE BRIEF PASSAGES IN A REVIEW.

FIRST EDITION

The author is grateful to the following publishers for permission to quote material as noted:

Dodd, Mead and Company; McGraw-Hill Ryerson Limited; and Ernest Benn, for lines from "Goodbye Little Cabin" in *Collected Poems of Robert Service.*

Alfred A. Knopf, Inc., for lines from "Henry King" in *Cautionary Verses* by Hilaire Belloc.

Photograph of "The Poole family in 1965" courtesy of Franklin Grant; "Freddie Gemmer, Sam and friends" courtesy of Guy Gannett Publishing Co.; "Sam, on the M.V. *Victoria*'s maiden voyage" courtesy of Andrew Wooden; photographs of Sam in the hospital courtesy of Judith Lachenmeyer; "Heart Transplant 120 with Stanford friend and the lady known as Claire" courtesy of San Francisco Antique Photo.

LIBRARY OF CONGRESS CATALOGING IN PUBLICATION DATA

Poole, Victoria.
  Thursday's child.

  1. Heart — Transplantation — Biography. 2. Poole, Sam. I. Title.
  RD598.P55 1979   617'.412 [B]   79-25767
  ISBN 0-316-71334-1

MV
Designed by Susan Windheim
Published simultaneously in Canada
by Little, Brown & Company (Canada) Limited

PRINTED IN THE UNITED STATES OF AMERICA

To three great institutions:
the heart transplant team at
Stanford University Medical Center,
Kent School,
and Sam

. . . Wednesday's child is full of woe,
Thursday's child has far to go . . .

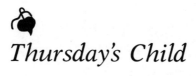

Thursday's Child

Prologue   Until this very moment I've always liked having a big family. I can't remember being bored or lonely. Bewildered, despairing, foul-tempered, yes, but bored or lonely, never. Right now, however, faced with telling a story about just one of my children, I could do without the unwieldy group of also-rans waiting in the wings. What's more, my literary endeavors have heretofore been limited to writing letters to the children, and as my only notable talent is for washing woodwork, "inadequate" is a word which floats often through my mind of late. Be that as it may . . .

In the halcyon days when having babies was no sin against mankind or the environment, my husband Parker and I had five in seven years and then, feeling abandonment at hand as we watched them grow, had a sixth to keep us company in our declining years. We also acquired a daughter-in-law, and a housekeeper who came "for a week" nineteen years ago, and they are family too. Add on my sister and her husband and daughter, who do everything with us, and the cast of characters swells to Russian-novel proportions.

3

Nor is it only in number that we are large. At five feet seven I am far shorter than everybody else, and the sight of the Poole family arriving en masse must strike terror into the heart of any hostess who collects spindly legged antiques or boasts a glass coffee table. Aside from that drawback, and immodest as it may sound, the children are most satisfactory. The eight of them (for Ruthie, the daughter-in-law, and Louise, the niece, are always ranked in position of age with ours, although they can't compete with Pooles for height) tolerate us adults kindly, organize us, and even seem to like to be with us.

The story is about Sam, our fifth child, who is currently a member of one of the most exclusive clubs in the world — but you will have to reach him in his proper order.

Malcolm is the oldest of our children. In the fall of 1975, when the story begins, he was twenty-four and quite dashing as an officer in the U.S. Coast Guard. He married Ruthie, whom he met on the first day of their first year at Trinity College in Hartford, Connecticut, and there would have been a family mutiny if he'd ever had another girl, for we all adored her on sight. Malcolm has always done well, been relatively good, and taken part in exotic things like rowing at the Henley Royal Regatta in England and sailing to Spain in transatlantic races.

When people ask, "Now, which is the one who fell in the cesspool?" they mean Pokie, our second son. In point of fact, he fell on it, not in it, from a tree, but in either case the results could not have been more drastic. Fourteen operations later, the loser in a battle with osteomyelitis, he was left with a bad left arm and hand and a determination to be wicked. Each gray hair and wrinkle in evidence upon his parents bears witness to the hair-raising schemes and adventures of his wild youth, and although Parker and I never doubted for a minute that Pokie would survive, we often wondered if we would. He eventually emerged from Tufts with an engineering degree, a true conservative's delight in his proper name — Parker Poole III — and a plan to become a millionaire by the time he was twenty-two. Twenty-three and still impecunious at the time of this story, he had extended his deadline to age twenty-five, and to that end he was enduring living at home with us, as an economy measure only.

Louise, the niece, is next in line. Not only beautiful but bright, she was twenty-two that fall, nine months younger than Pokie. Her academic career is a shining but unfollowed beacon in a sea of unstudious Pooles. She was left in our care one year just as school grades appeared in June. Parker opened all his own children's reports, making appropriate comments about each one's industry and effort, and then regarded Louise's. A's everywhere bewildered him for only a moment. "Well, Louise," he growled, impartial through and through, "what's this 'B' in guitar?"

Nine months younger again is Charlie. He watched his older brothers' careers carefully and evidently decided to shun most evils of adolescence, from pimples to arrests for illegal transportation of beer. To everyone's amazement he graduated from Kent School in Connecticut with honors and a gold medal for rowing with a victorious crew at Henley. A junior at Trinity in 1975, it seemed likely that he would depart from college in a similar blaze of glory.

Christina, the first of the Poole girls, two years younger than Charlie, terrified everyone by rapidly becoming six feet tall, but she did it with such grace that she was, and is, the toast of the playing fields and the dance floors. Incredibly messy, Tina is so filled with love and good cheer that even I, the dragon of the clean-up squad, wade through her room almost indulgently. Her three older brothers and her cousin made her early years a vale of tears, but now she is an indispensable part of the group. She followed Malcolm, Ruthie, Louise, and Charlie to Trinity, causing the family hymn to become "Five in five years, O bless-ed Trinity."

It is at this point that Sam, more properly Talcott Simes Poole, enters the picture. Almost seventeen, he was six feet two, ruggedly lean, and becoming, to his own pleasure, noticeably handsome. The only one of our children to resemble in any way my side of the family, he had inherited from my father the long, thin face of a medieval saint and heavy, drooping eyelids which were proving a great asset to his love life. His muscles and his sense of humor, however bad, interested him more, and only on rare occasions was there an indication that he might also have inherited Daddy's most unholy temper. There was certainly no indication at all that he was — as by accident of birth he happened to be — a Wednesday's child. "Full of woe" Sam was not. The fourth Poole to go to Kent, he was in the fifth form at the time.

The consolation of our declining years, Alexandra, concludes the group of children. Poor Alix — her entire eleven years had been spent being prodded, teased, and ordered about. Her school stories invariably began: "I have four brothers and a sister. I like my sister. My favorite brother is ———. She always cited the one who was at the moment farthest away and least in her hair.

It was when Sam was born that Dottie, our housekeeper, came for the week that has lasted nineteen years. I think that now Sam loves us equally, but when he was little I know he loved her more.

Dottie was the one who named him Sam. She used to take him with her to the supermarket.

"What a dear little boy," the checkout ladies would exclaim. "What's his name?"

"Talcott," Dottie would answer.

"What?" the ladies would ask.

"Talcott. T-A-L-C-O-T-T."

After several months of this she said "Sam" and ended the problem. "You and your fancy names," she sniffed at me, and Sam he remains.

My sister Rozzie, her husband Bill Richardson, Parker, and I are known even to ourselves as Aunt and Uncle. "Good morning, Aunt Roz," I say to her, or, "Hello, Uncle Bill — Uncle Parker wants to know where we are having the picnic today."

The Aunt and I, or the Snoop Sisters, as the children call us, grow to look and talk more alike as each day goes by. Rozzie, however, has vastly more élan and presence and, with only one daughter, vastly more available cash and fewer wrinkles. The wrinkles rankle because she is three years older. She is given to Auntie Mame moods during which she decides that nothing will do but a trip and sweeps off with Louise and any available Poole children to Bermuda, Wyoming, or Greece.

Her husband Bill is by birth a Philadelphian, by education a chemical engineer, and by inclination a Dixieland drummer. At my father's death, he had unwillingly become president of my family's fuel business, the A. R. Wright Company. With two college degrees and being from Philadelphia and all, Uncle Bill should add a degree of dignity to family life. He does not and, indeed, is invited to take part in all the children's activities, however nefarious.

At the end of this sea of people comes Parker Poole, upon whose large shoulders have fallen innumerable burdens. A friend of mine once asked me, "How could anyone as assy as you were when you were twenty-two have had the wit to find Parker?" I don't know, but it is indeed a miracle. Being friends with his children has never interested him in the slightest. He has been their father, and the fact that they want to talk to him and be with him surprises him not one bit. The children used to refer to him in the tones usually reserved for the Lord's Prayer as "Our Father." In between coping with his wife and offspring, he works with his brother Bill (universally called "Unkie" to distinguish him from Uncle Bill Richardson) at *his* family's salt-and-chemical business, the W. H. Shurtleff Company.

By the time December 1975 arrived, the children seemed to Parker and me and Bill and Rozzie to be the only uncomplicated things that had ever happened to us. My mother had died in November 1974 and my father the next June, at the age of eighty-six. To Rozzie and me, who had believed, as Daddy did himself, that he was immortal, it was a terrible confusion. The four of us were immersed in the grim complexities of becoming the "older generation": inheritances, lawyers, taxes, and too much real estate. Life became an endless Monopoly game.

Mother and Daddy spent their summers in a farmhouse at Cape Elizabeth, Maine, seven miles outside of Portland; Daddy had determined that Bill and Rozzie should inherit it. My parents also had a twenty-two-room red-brick winter house in Portland; Daddy declared it was made for Parker and me. Nervously awaiting bolts of lightning from up above or earthquakes from down below, we changed his plans. Rozzie and Bill already had an old farmhouse at Cape Elizabeth; they didn't want another, and even Daddy's wrath couldn't have induced me to move permanently into a twenty-two-room house. Parker and I volunteered to live in its vastness as caretakers until someone could be found to agree with Daddy that it was the best damned house in Portland and buy it. After that the Pooles would move permanently to my parents' summer house.

It took all the Yankee stoicism and practicality that Parker and I could muster to sell our own house in Portland, where all the children had grown up. We both had lumps in our throats as the movers drove off to their storage warehouse with our belongings and we moved three doors down the street to my parents', with only our bed and our kitchen table to remind us of our former independent state.

Rozzie would appear at our new abode daily, and the two of us dolefully worked away at the gloomy task of dividing and throwing out our parents' lives. Convinced that we would be emptying bureau drawers forever, and in a perpetual state of filth from crawling through attics and dark closets, we could hardly wait for the children to come home for Christmas and call a moratorium on estate settling.

Chapter One   The first time I noticed that
something was wrong with Sam was the day he came home
for Christmas vacation. Dottie, our housekeeper, says, regularly and accusingly, "I told you he was sick in September
when he went back to school." When I remind her that he
had seen a doctor and been given a clean bill of health less
than a week before fall term started, she is not impressed.

That's neither here nor there, though. The first time I noticed was on Thursday, December 18, the winter we stayed
at my parents' house.

Parker made the long, five-hour drive to Kent to fetch
Sam home on Wednesday. It was normally a dreaded excursion, but Parker had grown to love the Christmas trip.
He spent the night with Hart Perry, the dean of boys,
and his family, went to the Episcopal chapel service, and
always came home exuding goodwill toward men and
church schools, staunch unpracticing Congregationalist
that he is.

Charlie and Tina were driving home together from Trinity that Thursday too, but it was a foregone conclusion that

Sam and Parker would reach Portland first. As Charlie had said gloomily Sunday night on the telephone, "Tina always forgets things, and we have to go back."

At home I worked valiantly at decking the halls. All the children — with the exception of Pokie, whose baronial tastes comprehended magnificence — had confided to me at Thanksgiving, "It's going to be weird being in that house for Christmas, Mum," and in truth they'd been to more funerals than festivities in it. There was no way I could make it look like home, but I was at least determined that it would look the way it did at Christmas before Mother got sick. The downstairs windows and the front door had their wreaths, and garlands were more or less symmetrically entwined around the four pillars on the front porch. I'd even exhumed the lights Mother always put in the windows.

At one o'clock, delighted with the effects of my efforts, I was making a final housewifely check of Sam and Charlie's room on the third floor when I heard the front door burst open and Sam call, "Hi, Mum, I'm home!"

I tore down the stairs, and by the time I reached the second floor he was yelling, "I got my varsity letter!"

I called back, "Great. Oh, I'm glad you're home," as I ran down the last flight to the front hall, but halfway down I stopped dead in my tracks. Before my eyes was rummage-sale day at the high-school gymnasium. I could only hope that my parents' normally impressive front hall was still alive and well buried somewhere beneath the avalanche of Sam's belongings. Two ancient Chinese chairs that Mother never let us touch, let alone put anything on, groaned under the weight of his impedimenta. Muddy cleats, hockey skates, and evil-looking "sweats" topped a more anonymous heap of sports coats and sweaters. On the floor a complete stereo system, grimy laundry bags, and sticks for every imaginable sport competed with Moriah, our German shepherd, and her welcoming tail for the last inch of space.

There was a wide, low railing that edged the last landing of the staircase. Rozzie and I used to jump over it when we were children, but I found it took courage to do that now, though it still made a splendid repository for the mail and hats and coats. Sam was standing at it, burrowing down into a huge tan backpack precariously perched on the edge.

"Don't you dare open that down here, Sam Poole," I shrieked at him, running down the rest of the stairs.

"But my varsity letter's in it, Mum," he protested. "We had the football banquet last night, and you're looking at old Number Seventy-one." He straightened up, flexing both arms over his head in his favorite Muhammad Ali "I am the greatest" pose, and the mess was forgotten.

He didn't look like old Number 71 to me. Marley's Ghost would have been more like it. His face was gaunt and his eyes had retreated somewhere into the back of his head. There were dark circles underneath them and his eyelids were not in the least romantic. They drooped so low that he was peering up at me from underneath them, and he'd lost pounds since Thanksgiving.

"Sam," I gasped, "what's happened to you? Didn't you even go to bed during exams?"

He hadn't, according to Parker, who was just coming in the front door with a last load of Sam's possessions. "He's been working too hard," he stated emphatically. "It's fine to do well on your exams, Sam, but you've got to learn to pace yourself. You'll be a dead hero if you keep on at this rate. I've told him he's got to get some rest," he said to me. "And he's still got that cold he had at Thanksgiving. He coughed all the way home in the car."

In itself this speech was unusual, for normally all Parker says when he comes home from a trip in the middle of the day is, "Well, I've got to get back to the office." After he left I turned back to regard Sam with an even more critical eye. "Is it the same cold, Sam," I asked, "or another one?"

He was still digging down in the pack, heaving out underwear and socks with abandon. "I don't know," he said. "It isn't really a cold. It's just I cough all the time," and then he started coughing, as if to prove the point.

Coughs are not rarities on my side of the family, nor are they alarming in general. Along with Rozzie and me, Sam had inherited the "Simes cough," which is deep and loose and mostly, to the despair of our husbands, nocturnal. It lasts for months after the first sniffle appears, so the fact that Sam had been coughing for the three weeks since Thanksgiving didn't bother me a bit. What did bother me was that he was having an attack in the middle of the day that ought only to come in the middle of the night. The cough itself had an unfamiliar sound. It sloshed. As if floodgates were open in his chest, whatever massive amount of mucus he coughed up into his throat seemed instantly to be replaced by more. You could hear it rumbling in.

It didn't seem to bother Sam, though. He kept on with his exploration of the backpack and eventually emerged from its interior with the gray felt *K* edged with blue. "How about that after being out all last season with my knee?" he exulted. "I really worked for it, Mum."

"It's nice, dear," I said. Being totally uncoordinated myself, I don't really understand sports, and anyway I'd seen varsity letters before. Like all proper Pooles, Sam would have more than his share by the time he graduated from Kent in a year and a half.

14

His face told me that "nice" was not enough. I collected myself and tried again.

"It's absolutely great, Sam. I simply couldn't be prouder of you, but" — I couldn't forbear another second — "that cough is terrible. I'm going to call Dr. Mansfield. Would you get all your junk up to the third floor and the dirty things down to the cellar before Charlie and Tina get home with theirs and the house turns into a pumpkin?"

"Okay," he said, "but make the appointment for the end of vacation. I don't want it to mess up my skiing." Before unpacking the debris, however, he gave a horrendous from-the-bottom-of-the-barrel huck that started in the back of his throat, drained his nose, and brought up God knows what from his chest.

"That's revolting, Sam," I said, promptly turning back to him. "It was all right when you were in the eighth grade, and I know you have a cold, but you're too old to make noises like that."

Injured, he gazed at me with the same expression he'd been wearing since the eighth grade whenever "couth" was discussed between us. "You don't want me to keep all that gunk down there, do you?" he said. "Dottie says it's good to get it up," and, hoisting his stereo speakers under his arms, he proceeded to drag his way up the stairs.

I stood in front of the landing, defeated, watching his progress. There are forty-four steps from the first floor to the third in my parents' house. And twenty more from the first floor to the cellar, I'd learned in the course of the past three months. They'd done wonders for my wind, but Sam was going up them as slowly and despondently as some of Mother's ancient maids, who would wheeze and groan their way up and down for a week or so and then give their notice.

15

Well, I thought, it certainly wasn't speed that made him old Number 71, and I started to laugh, remembering what Hart Perry had said about him during Parents' Weekend in October. "The rest of the team we time with a stopwatch," he'd drawled, "but for Sam we just turn over the egg timer."

His remark had already become a family joke, but, standing at the foot of the stairs, I suddenly remembered that Sam had had a cold that weekend too.

My God, I thought, he's had a cold all fall, and I went into Daddy's office, a dark-paneled little room just to the right of the front door, and called the doctor.

"January fifth," the nurse announced, "at ten o'clock."

I was just thanking her and hanging up when down the stairs roared Sam. He tore open the front door with a blood-curdling howl, and I heard Alix wailing from the porch, "Mummeeee, make him stop."

It was comforting. He can't be all that sick, I said to myself as I watched poor Al trying to dodge past him into the front hall.

By the time everyone got home that night, Sam's condition was forgotten in the general confusion. Tina had a dreadful cold, which I promptly caught, and the whole house reverberated with hacks and sneezes. In the seasonal bedlam, no one even brought up Sam's morning habits until the day before Christmas. Tina, Alix, the dog, and I were all in the big living room. Alix was wrapping presents, Moriah was sleeping, and I was drifting vaguely through the room with a duster in preparation for the next day's festivities. Tina was making Uncle Bill's Christmas present, a Fourth of July toasting book for the upcoming Bicentennial. It appeared from the number of pages that quantity rather than quality was the determining factor in her selection of patriots.

I'd just looked over her shoulder and commented — "You'll all be sloshed by the time you get to Paul Revere's horse" — when we heard the dire noises that regularly heralded Sam's morning advent: the thudding of slow, heavy feet, huckings and gurglings, coughs and unspat spit. They meant that he had completed his "hour shower" and that the hot-water system was sabotaged for the rest of the day.

"That damn Sam," I groaned. "He's getting worse and worse."

"He's disgusting, Mummy," Alix complained, while into the living room dragged Sam. He was barefoot and barechested, his dungarees sagged at half-mast, and wet, tangled hair streamed down over his face. No good-mornings, no smile. He crossed the room, tripped over the dog, changed Alix's TV program over her protests, and collapsed in Mother's most comfortable armchair.

"He's like the pig in *Alice in Wonderland*," I said to Alix. " 'He only does it to annoy, because he knows it teases.' " Sam's comment was another gurgling huck, which I ignored. Unlike the rest of us, he was always a late and sullen riser, but in the course of the morning, having invented a game to prove to his delight and to Alix's dismay that the dog liked everyone better than her, he rejoined the human race.

"Mum, I don't see how Sam ever gets to classes at Kent," Tina said to me later in the day. "It takes him longer and longer every day to get functioning. Maybe he's got mono again." (Sam had electrified us all by having mononucleosis at age three. It was such a classic case — involving even a rash, which is rare — that our pediatrician brought all his hospital students to view him. It had been very unnerving having all those white coats and stethoscopes flailing around the bedroom.)

"I don't think it could be, Tina," I said. "When he had mono, he had a fever all the time, and he doesn't have any now. I think he's just dragged out from fall term and exams." But it was beginning to cross my mind that after a week at home he should be looking better.

The next day at Christmas dinner, though, he was as chipper as a lark. No sooner had we sat down fourteen strong at the table than he rose to his feet, resplendent in his green blazer and combed hair, and clanked his knife against his wineglass. (Underneath the table I knew his feet were encased in the grungy Adidas that seemed, like some rare fungus, to have attached themselves to his extremities. Still, from the waist up he was splendid.) It was entirely possible to believe that he was going to make a proper Christmas toast, and Parker's brother Bill and his wife Dana gave him their courteous attention. The rest of us groaned. It was "drunk count" time.

Every Christmas morning for years, Pokie and Sam set off ostensibly to replenish the ice supply. The true purpose of their excursion, however, was to take a head count of holiday drunks at the local bus station and to disrupt Christmas dinner with the annual report.

This year Louise said firmly, "Down, boy," as I moaned, "Oh, Sam, not today," and several family members booed. Looking aggrieved, Sam sat down meekly. Nonetheless, by the end of dinner we'd heard in detail, as we knew we would, about each and every one.

Painful as it is to admit, the general tenor of conversation at our Christmas dinner table was hardly more elevating. Nostalgia was the theme. Unkie claimed he had heard Daddy roar, "Where the hell is the son of a bitch?" at Mother's funeral when the clergyman didn't appear. Uncle Bill told a mesmerized Dana about his plan — foiled when the undertaker got to the house first — to stuff and mechanize Daddy so he could smoke, curse, and pound on his desk into perpetuity. Rozzie and I cheerfully recalled that the last time we'd sat at the dining-room table was the day Daddy died.

The thought itself was sobering, however, and Rozzie and I toasted our dead parents with tears in our eyes and the past with more tears in our eyes, at which point Bill and Parker told us to be quiet.

Ruthie drank to surviving her first Poole Christmas. Malcolm, who had had the duty on Governors Island in New York Harbor on Christmas Eve and had driven all night to get home, toasted his own swift separation from the Coast Guard. Unkie drank to the day when Malcolm could come to work at the W. H. Shurtleff Company, which caused Uncle Bill to insist that, although he had Pokie at A. R. Wright already, it would be his turn when Charlie came along, and Sam demanded loudly to know who got him.

"Someone very unlucky," Louise said, fixing him with a scathing glance.

What with toastings and reminiscences, Rozzie and I didn't get to the kitchen until after five. The children had put the first load in the dishwasher and departed, according to our rule. We know they think we are inefficient, and we don't like them to watch us. (Ruthie, entering the family, asked with horror, "But how can it take anyone three hours to wash the dishes?" We don't know, but it does — and sometimes even longer. It depends on how much we have to discuss.)

By six thirty we'd gotten to the pots. Rozzie was at the sink meticulously scrubbing the spinach saucepan, and I was unloading the dishwasher. We'd established that the children planned to go to Sugarloaf Mountain, where we ski, the next morning, which was Friday, that she and I would go up with Alix and the dogs the following Tuesday, and that the fathers could drive up together on Wednesday, New Year's Eve.

We'd covered the love lives of the children who were old enough to have them, and then I said, really for lack of anything better to say, "You know, Rozzie, I wish I'd made the doctor's appointment for Sam for before he goes skiing. He's had that cold all fall and he doesn't look right."

"I know," she said, "I think he has some dreadful disease — like leukemia." Rozzie has always been called Cassandra in the family, but I'd never heard her say anything like that before. I jerked my head up out of the dishwasher. She was calmly scrubbing away at a pot.

"Rozzie, that's a terrible thing to say," I said, and then, after a moment's thought, I added triumphantly: "Anyway, you don't cough with leukemia, you get sores on your legs."

Rozzie never admits she's wrong, but she did have the grace to admit that even she had never before connected that particular symptom to that particular disease. We dropped the subject and pottered on amicably, and by the time I woke up the next morning I had a whole new batch of worries.

The day after Christmas is my birthday. As we had surmised, it saw the departure of all properly mature children (with the exception of Ruth and Malcolm, who had to go back to Governors Island and the Coast Guard) for our ski camps at Sugarloaf Mountain, three hours north of Portland by car. The Lord honored the day with a dreadful ice storm, and I felt not one but twenty years older as I watched a section of the battered fleet of Poole automobiles start off.

Pokie and Sam traveled together in the former's "double Datsun," whose green front end and tan rear represented the marriage of two wrecked ones. Charlie, always independent, departed alone in his ancient Volkswagen.

Louise took Christina in her car, to my relief. She had a relatively sound machine, being, as her mother puts it, "the spoiled only child." Although poor Louise actually has had little opportunity to enjoy such a status, having had to share everything with the Pooles since birth, her sturdy car was initially a comfort to me that morning. Standing on the front porch that only partially protected me from the pelting sleet, however, I soon decided it was not enough. We were crazy to say any of them could go, let alone Sam with that cold, I thought, as I retreated into the house. If they ever get to Sugarloaf in this weather, what's going to happen to him in those camps?

In 1958, the year that Sam was born, Sugarloaf was a new ski development. Fifteen miles of timberland separated it in both directions from the nearest two towns. There were no inns, no chalets, and certainly no condominiums then, and that fall Parker found a veritable treasure. Just feet from the entrance to the mountain road were four old cabins — always called "camps" in Maine — which had belonged to a lumber company. For an annual rental of $150 (the price has now soared to $250), he was given his choice of the entire bunch. Parker firmly maintains that he selected our camp because it had the best exposure and ignores rude remarks about "choices" and "rotten eggs," but aside from exposure there is little else to recommend it. It has no water or electricity, its floors sag alarmingly, but it is ours. It is called Camp Bruin in honor of the bear Parker shot nearby. The neighboring cabin, which has been resurrected enough to house Pokie and his army of friends, is known for obvious reasons as Camp Ruin.

The "veritable treasure" aspect of the camps has faded somewhat for me, but during the turmoils of the sixties the children never once accused us of having false values. I expect that's some comfort as we split our wood, haul our water from a frozen river, and yearn for baths.

Rozzie and I long ago admitted to each other, however, that nobody ever gets over anything in either of the camps. Whatever therapeutic value mountain air is supposed to have, it loses it once transmitted through the walls of Bruin and Ruin. Pokie called on Monday to confirm that truth.

The occasion for the call was the "we're out of" list, but somewhere between kerosene and paper towels he interrupted himself to say, "Mother, I don't think Sam's too well. I'm kind of worried about him."

The fact that Pokie rarely worries out loud and never to his mother was cause for alarm, and my heart sank. However, balanced against the anguish of Why did I let Sam go? was the sure knowledge that I could never have kept him at home. He hadn't had a fever; he had a cough. Tina had a cough and she was going; I had a cough and I certainly wasn't staying home because of it. Rozzie and I had been brought up with such care by Mother after our sister died of "mastoid" that we were bundled and swaddled and thrown into bed for the slightest malaise. It made us healthy indeed, but it left me with an abiding loathing for rubbers and overshoes, hot-water bottles, medicines, and coddling in general. The long lisle stockings I had to wear when everyone else was in ankle socks and the sniffle that cost me my part in *Robin Hood* had forged a medical philosophy that let feverless children do pretty much what they felt like doing. It had withstood the test of time and six children until it met Sam and his cough.

"Is it the cough, Pokie?" I asked.

"Well, it's that too, but mostly he just seems worn out. He didn't ski yesterday, and he stayed at Ruin all day."

Dear God, I thought, what can be wrong with him?

Somehow at night with a cozy fire in the airtight stove, you don't notice the ceilings festooned with black cobwebs, and the buzzing of warmed-up flies behind the streaked paper walls seems rather soothing. Even the outhouse becomes endurable after a drink or two. But to spend an entire day in either camp by choice, you'd have to be sick beyond caring.

"Does he have a temperature now?" I asked.

The answer was still an unequivocal no, and the only clue Pokie could offer to Sam's peculiar condition was the cough syrup our family swears by. "He took a double dose Saturday," he said, "and almost passed out skiing. He's been taking a lot of it."

Relief flooded over me. "Why didn't you say so before?" I said. "That stuff is lethal. No wonder he couldn't ski yesterday. Be sure you tell him it's just one teaspoon twice a day," I told him, and we returned to our quartermastering.

Tina and Louise told us that Sam was taking a nap at Ruin when Rozzie and I got to Sugarloaf on Tuesday afternoon, and, grabbing armloads of grocery bags out of our car, they ushered us through Bruin's front door. Entering

Bruin at any time of year is a shock to the system, but the first arrival of the season is stupefying. You are in the living room, and, because terminal settling is in progress, you have to walk downhill through it to get to the kitchen. You walk uphill across the kitchen to get to the outhouse, but when you first get to Camp Bruin you don't walk anywhere. You stand rooted to the spot, as Rozzie and I always do, hoping it's a bad dream that will go away.

Behind the airtight stove, the red wooden toilet seat hung on its accustomed nail, warming for the next trip to the outhouse. Encouragingly decorated by Uncle Bill with sprays of painted buttercups and daisies, the seat added the only touch of color to a room where all else was soot-smudged gray, but the thought of its ultimate destination wasn't encouraging at all. Ruthie, a proper Bostonian, had emphatically stated on her first trip to Bruin, "I will nevah evah put that thing over my arm right in front of people and go to that outhouse." Although time and the demands of nature shortly made her less adamant, as it had Rozzie and me, I knew just how she felt.

We were still regarding the pure unadulterated squalor of the living room with dismay when Sam appeared in the doorway with his best friend, Freddie Gemmer.

They were in great spirits. The older children had appointed Sam the host of the annual New Year's Eve party at Ruin. It was no real honor, because everybody's friends came, and all it really meant was that the one whose party it had been declared was burdened on New Year's morning with cleanup and complaints. Sam, however, had evidently already proved to his own and Fred's satisfaction that he was equal to the task.

Going up the mountain in the gondola that afternoon, according to Freddie, "a very average Joe" that neither of them had ever seen before had said to Sam, "Hey, man, you makin' the scene at Sam Poole's on New Year's Eve?"

"I started to crack up," Freddie said, "but Sam just sat there. He put on his shades and said, 'Hey, man, you read the plot wrong. There's no scene there. Sam got busted,' and the guy was so dumb he bought it."

Sam's cool had deserted him only when they emerged from the gondola. "He started laughing so hard," Freddie said, convulsed all over again, "he dropped his cigarette inside his parka and couldn't stop laughing to get it out."

Rozzie and I looked at the two of them, shaking our heads. They both had on identical orange parkas, and stray wisps of down were indeed escaping from a large hole in the front of Sam's, but that wasn't the only difference I noticed. Freddie looked healthy and his parka was becoming. Against Sam's pale face the bright orange looked garish, and for the first time in the fourteen years that they'd been up to no good together, I thought with surprise, Why, Freddie looks bigger than Sam.

The afternoon had had a tonic effect on Sam's spirits, however, and I resolved to avoid looking at him in the parka. By suppertime he had identified the "average Joe" of the gondola as the kind of guy who drives around in 90-degree heat with his car windows up so the world will think he has air conditioning. By the next afternoon, when the fathers arrived, poor Joe had sunk so low he was accused of going to French restaurants and ordering *"la même chose"* to show he understood the menu. Sam was still gloating about him as he set off to host the New Year's Eve bash at Ruin, which appeared to be its usual back-to-back and belly-to-belly success.

In the morning, however, we were eating breakfast at the kitchen table at Bruin when Sam suddenly appeared in the doorway like a specter. His face was ashen and he was coughing.

"Where's a broom?" he asked the room at large between hacks. "I gotta clean up."

"How about some eggs, Sambo?" Bill asked him.

He shook his head. "No, thanks, Uncle Bill. I'm not very hungry."

With our broom and dustpan in hand he slowly started out the door to go back to Ruin, and the whole first morning of the New Year was haunted by the shuffle of a pale sick Sam, dragging his way laboriously back and forth between the two camps, a sorry ghost of his noisy old self.

He brightened up only once, when Rozzie asked him to explain a joke she'd heard the night before and didn't understand.

"Aunt Roz," he said with a wicked smile, "you're not old enough," but the effort started him coughing and he fell back into a chair. He sat there hunched over with his head almost between his knees, clutching his sides while his whole body strained and shook with the spasm.

"Sam, you've got to go home," Parker said. "You'll never get over that up here."

He didn't even protest at missing the revels the other children had planned for the next few days and drove back to Portland with Parker, Alix, a friend of hers, and me. "Thank God he's going to the doctor Monday," I kept saying to myself all the way home in the car.

By Monday, though, the cough was again just a cough, and when Sam set off for his appointment with the doctor a little before ten, I'd forgotten most of my panic.

"Be sure to come right back," I said to him as he went

out the front door. "You've got a million things to do before you go back to school on Wednesday."

He didn't. I waited and I wondered, and at noon I called Alice Gemmer, Freddie's mother. Fred was missing too. We decided they'd gone off together to escape us and really didn't much blame them. Ten minutes later the phone rang.

"This is Tom Mansfield," said the familiar voice of our family doctor. "I didn't hear anything in Sam's chest, but I sent him over to the hospital for a routine chest X-ray. He's on his way home now, but they called me from there to say that his heart is badly enlarged."

I stood there in Daddy's office, holding the phone and saying nothing for what seemed like ages. As absurd as it is, the only thing I can remember thinking was, What if he can't row in the spring?

I finally must have collected myself, for I can hear myself asking Dr. Mansfield if he meant an "athlete's heart." One of Sam's friends had had one. "They decided it was perfectly normal for someone who exercised a lot," I said. "Sam's been playing football all fall and he went out for crew last spring. Don't you think that's what it is?"

He didn't, but on the other hand he didn't think that the enlargement was caused by a congenital condition. "It would have showed up before now," he said. "It's my bet that the problem is caused by a virus infection connected with this cold he has." In that case, he explained, Sam's heart would gradually go back to normal as the virus subsided, if he did nothing in the meantime to strain it. He had seen something like this only once before — in a middle-aged man whose heart was as grossly enlarged as Sam's. "In a year," he said consolingly, "you'd never have known from the X-rays that he had had a problem."

I was still gulping at the "year" when he threw out a word of caution that terrified me. The enlargement could also have been caused by a past viral infection, in which case the heart would never be normal again. It could have been a strep throat; it could have been just a cold; it could have been almost anything.

"Could it have been mono?" I asked, racking my brain to recall all Sam's childhood diseases.

"It's hard to tell," he said, "because we have nothing to compare today's X-ray with. If we had an earlier one to check it against, we'd have a better idea. Has he ever had a chest X-ray before that you know of?"

"No," I answered, and my voice sounded strangely divorced from me. "No, I don't think so, but, Tom, you don't think rowing could have caused it, do you?"

He was too kind to say "I just told you that we don't know," and instead went on to list what must be done next. Sam should not go back to Kent, nor should he do anything that might strain his heart until he had seen a cardiologist. "And that's the problem right now," he said. "Those guys are so busy it's hard to get an appointment right off the bat." He would try to set up something and call me back later in the afternoon, but I was to be sure that Sam understood he must not exercise. No, he did not have to go to bed and, yes, he could drive a car, but no exercise.

As he was about to hang up, I suddenly remembered why Sam had gone to see him in the first place. "But what about the cough?" I asked. "Does it have anything to do with his heart?"

Again there was no sure answer. The cough, however, was not to be suppressed; it was to be expectorated, and he had told Sam what cough medicine he should use. "And," he finished, "I think all your other kids who haven't had a chest X-ray ought to. Let me know when they're around, and we'll make appointments for them."

"Thank you," I said, "I will," and I hung up. I felt numb and stupid. I stood at my father's desk doing absolutely nothing until I suddenly remembered that Dr. Mansfield had said that Sam was on his way home from the hospital. The hospital, where we all go for everything, was only four blocks from the house and Sam had a car. He should be here by now. What was I going to tell him?

I've got to call Parker, I thought, but suddenly it came over me that I had to get out of that room. The sun never penetrated Daddy's office. He had always had a roaring fire going, which cheered it up and brightened the dark mahogany of the walls, but there was no fire in it now, and the room was cold and full of ghosts. I didn't want to be there when Sam came in, and I fled upstairs to call Parker and wait.

Chapter Two

Crisis makes me even more disheveled than usual. If it weren't for a New England conscience, which doesn't keep you from doing wrong but keeps you from enjoying it, I would say that a majestic — almost divinely inspired — calm swept over me as I went up the stairs, but it didn't.

When I found that Parker had left the office for lunch, I only said "Damn" and slammed down the receiver, but after that I fell apart. I started running wildly from bedroom to bedroom, making beds that were already made, pulling up shades that were already pulled up, and cursing. In Pokie's room I cursed poor old Matthew, Mark, Luke, and John, who were carved on the massive oak headboard of the bed, for their lack of concern with my problems, and in ours I cursed myself for never being dressed when disaster struck. Somehow it seemed absolutely necessary that I should be before Sam got home, but it became a staggeringly difficult task.

I couldn't find my toothbrush. (Of course he had a bad

heart with a mother who couldn't even get dressed in the morning and had never had him have a chest X-ray.)

My blue jeans had vanished. (Well, the doctors should decide when someone needs an X-ray. X-rays aren't mothers' responsibilities. And what did he mean, "Have the other kids had one?")

That question produced a terrifying picture of six wet and dripping X-rays, hanging side by side from their metal clips, exhibiting six enlarged hearts. To obliterate it I stood, stark naked in the middle of the bedroom, wailing ungrammatically at no one, "Oh, where the hell is Sam? Why is no one where I want them when I need them?"

I was still unhinged and undressed when I heard the front door open. Grabbing my bathrobe, I ran to the head of the stairs.

"Sam! Sam, is that you?" I yelled.

He was just coming in from the vestibule that separated the front hall from the outdoors. Stray wisps of goose down were still seeping out of the cigarette burn in his orange parka, and he had his blue ski hat, his dark-glasses case, and his ski gloves in one hand. The other was fiercely extracting a cigarette from his mouth.

"Christ," he said before I could speak, "that frigging hospital! I've been there since ten thirty having one goddamned chest X-ray after another. 'Go out and wait.' 'Come in and have another.' 'Go out and wait.' " He mimicked the voice of all unwanted authority. "I must have had seven before they told me to go home. Well, I didn't go home either," he added with satisfaction. "I just sat in the car and smoked."

"Sam," I said, from the top of the stairs. "Dr. Mansfield just called, and you can't go back to school yet."

He was standing in front of the railing at the foot of the

stairs, just where he had stood when he came home for vacation with his football letter. He stared disbelievingly at me for a second and then slammed the hat, the glasses case, and the gloves down on the railing. I will never forget that sound. It was identical to the one my father made when he crashed his fist on his desk, and it terrified me. It took me a second to realize that it was my son and not my father I was crossing.

"Sam, listen," I said hesitantly (I could never have said anything at all to Daddy). "Listen, Dr. Mansfield says your heart is enlarged. That's what all the X-rays were about, and you can't go back to school until you've seen a cardiologist. He's trying to get you an appointment now."

His anger passed as quickly as it came, and he started to smile. "Aw, come on, Mum," he said. "What's the joke? I'm fine."

"Oh, darling," I said, running down the stairs and putting my arms around him, "I'm not joking, but I know it will be nothing. Dr. Mansfield says it's probably just a virus, but they've got to be sure."

I rattled on, reminding him of his friend with the athlete's heart. "Just think about Malcolm Tisdale," I said. "He was back playing lacrosse just as soon as the doctors decided that's what it was."

He cheered up. After reminding me that fifth-form year was when you had to get everything going for you, and you couldn't miss school, he took a last drag of his cigarette and asked if Freddie had called.

"No," I said. "Mrs. Gemmer's lost him too. He went to Dr. Rothmore's at ten, and she hasn't seen him since."

"Whaddaya think they decided he's got?" he demanded scornfully and announced that he was departing in order to find out.

He went into Daddy's office and called Hart Perry at Kent before he left.

"Hi, Mr. Perry. This is Sam," I heard him say, as cheerfully as though he'd just won a crew race. "Yeah, Sam Poole. Oh, we're all great. We had a great Christmas, but, Mr. Perry, some dumb doctors up here think there's something wrong with my heart, and I can't come back on Wednesday."

There was quiet while he listened to Hart, and then he burst out laughing. "Okay, Mr. Perry, I won't. See ya," and he hung up. Dropping his voice into Hart's low, slow growl, he said to me, "Mr. Perry says, 'Well, don't let it interfere with your rowing, Sam,' " and he went out the front door.

By the time he came back, Parker had called me and put, as he always does, a Poole calm over my Simes despair. It was comforting to have someone else know, and, reassured, I even managed to get myself dressed.

From some dark recess of my mind, I dredged up the story of my Great-Aunt Pauline, whose X-rays at Johns Hopkins got confused with those of a terminal cancer patient. After many months of excellent physical health but extreme mental anguish, the error was unearthed, and Aunt Pauline died forty-seven years later at the age of one hundred and three. Even though a similar error seemed unlikely in a modern hospital, it gave me something to hope for while I tried to get back to my chores.

I was changing sheets in Sam and Charlie's room on the third floor when I heard boots clumping up the stairs amid raucous laughter and realized that Sam and Freddie had finally been reunited.

"You think I've got troubles, Mum," Sam exploded as they came into the room. "Wait'll you hear what happened to Fred. Dr. Rothmore said he has hemorrhoids and made him go to the hospital for an enema."

Tom Mansfield called back at about four thirty. "I can't find anyone who can see him for three weeks," he stated flatly.

"Well, he says he'll keep trying," I reported to Parker on the phone, "but it's one hell of a note when you've lived in Portland for generations and can't even get a lousy doctor's appointment. He can't miss all that school, and he's got achievement tests for college too. God, if he doesn't have a heart problem now, he'll get one worrying by the time he's waited at home for three weeks."

Parker is by nature slow to anger, and his response was noncommittal, but the half hour between my call and the closing of the W. H. Shurtleff Company gave him just the right amount of time to simmer up to a boil. He strode into the kitchen, where Sam was dolefully relating to Pokie the events of the "frigging hospital," without even a hello.

"That Morris kid," he said to Sam, "the one from Portland who goes to Kent. Isn't her father a heart man?"

Sam had been sitting hunched dejectedly over the kitchen table, aimlessly weaving the salt and pepper shakers back and forth in front of him, ever since Tom Mansfield's call. At Parker's question he looked up with positive delight and the old "Our Father" awe.

"God, Dad, would you call him?" he asked.

"You're damned right I will," Parker exploded, purposefully chomping on a large piece of pilot bread as he headed off for the telephone in Daddy's office.

I looked at his departing back with admiration, and, with unaccustomed affection, at the trail of crumbs he left behind him. Ed Morris was a cardiac surgeon, not a cardiologist. With a daughter at Kent, though, he'd certainly realize that missing three weeks would be tantamount to throwing the whole year down the drain and find someone who would be willing to check Sam out.

"He says it would be a disaster," Parker reported with satisfaction as he came back to the kitchen. "He's going to get Dr. George Hall, a cardiologist at the hospital, to look at him right away, even though he doesn't usually see private patients. Tom Mansfield will let us know tomorrow when and at what time."

It was everything we'd wanted, but somehow I felt offended. "Damn," I said. "Why is it always 'It's not what you know, but who you know'? What if you didn't know anybody?"

"No," Parker said, "it's not that. It's 'If you want something done, do it yourself.' "

On Thursday morning at nine o'clock, Parker drove Sam back to the hospital. The X-ray Department was bypassed for Cardiology, on the eighth floor, where an echogram and electrocardiogram had been scheduled by Dr. Hall.

I used the time while they were gone to try to regroup. Since Monday night, life with the Pooles could best be described as a zoo, in the children's vernacular. It had been impossible to concentrate on anyone's problems, let alone Sam's heart. Two interior decorators arrived from New York in a snowstorm on Tuesday morning, loaded with samples, order blanks, and smiles. In the chaos of Monday, I had entirely forgotten that I had asked them to come to help with my parents' summer house, the one which would ultimately become the Poole homestead. Christina and Charlie and Charlie's girl reappeared from Sugarloaf, and there was no Dottie to housekeep. Following the pattern of a year in which Murphy's Law — "If anything can possibly go wrong, it will" — had proved infallible, she had taken a leave of absence in early December to have her gallbladder removed.

When she heard about Sam on Monday night, she was bound and determined to ignore her doctor's orders and return to work the next day.

"You can't," I said. "Anyway, it wasn't my cooking that enlarged his heart," but I could plainly tell that she did not agree. It took me more than an hour to convince her that Sam was safe without her for at least a few more days.

Meanwhile, bedlam reigned supreme and the laundry piled high in the cellar. Between icy forays with me to my parents' summer house to measure floor space and wall space, the interior decorators ate without complaint with us in the kitchen, where conversation bypassed wallpapers and swatches to deal exclusively with Sam's condition. They didn't once object to Moriah, who shed all over their black New York suits. They even tried valiantly to sort out Tina and Alix from Charlie's girl, and Sam from Charlie and Pokie, but it was a losing battle.

I was so bewildered by the time Parker escorted them to the airport Wednesday night that I didn't even correct them when they said, "We hope Peter's heart won't be anything serious."

"He'll be fine," I murmured, and even the relative peace of Thursday morning did little to put me back in working order.

It was well after noon when Sam and Parker reappeared in the front hall. One look at their faces and my heart sank.

"There's no mistake," Parker said. "I talked to Dr. Hall after the tests, and the 'echo' confirms everything. Tom

Mansfield will give us a full report this afternoon at his office."

He put his hand on Sam's shoulder and smiled. "Cheer up, Sammy. You get rid of the cough, and I bet the whole thing will clear up. At least Dr. Hall said you could go back to school, so that's something. You've got to look on the bright side."

He is worried, I thought as he gave me my I've-got-to-get-back-to-the-office kiss and started out the door. I'd never heard him call Sam "Sammy" before, and with Parker any change in address spells deep concern. (When I become "Victoria," it means I'm talking too much again.) The old olive green coat he wears in the winter, with the hood dangling down the back from a solitary button, looked as tired as he did. One hand on the doorknob, he turned around.

"Remember, Sam. Dr. Hall said no more smoking."

I walked the three blocks to Dr. Mansfield's office alone that afternoon. Sam didn't want to come. The "don'ts" and "no mores" were obviously beginning to rankle. "I've got to pack," he said. "Just find out what I can do."

I met Parker in the waiting room, and we barely had time to sit down before Tom appeared in the doorway.

"C'mon in," he said, peering at us over the top of his steel-rimmed spectacles.

Tom Mansfield's office is as unpretentious and straight-forward as he is, and so small that he has to swing side-ways in his swivel chair to face you. No one ever emerged from it saying, "I think my gastrointestinal disorder paid for that new Oriental rug."

"Things don't look so hot," he said. "Even though his cardiogram is still pretty normal, his heart isn't."

"But why couldn't it be an athlete's heart?" I protested. Nothing if not dogged, I freely admit to Parker's accusation that I beat dead horses. I had tracked down the full story of Sam's friend. He had been permanently pulled off the playing fields until a cardiologist at Children's Hospital in Boston suggested that a heart catheterization be done. The results proved that the heart was indeed large, but that the enlargement was normal. "How can you decide that Sam's isn't normal without doing a catheterization?" I finished.

The echogram seemed to be the answer. It was a new device, Tom explained, and could detect a heart condition by sound waves quite as accurately and with considerably less risk, pain, and commotion. With a so-called athlete's heart, enlargement comes from the strong wall of muscle that builds evenly around the heart. Sam's echogram proved conclusively that his heart wall was very weak, the enlargement very abnormal.

"We suspected right on Monday," he said. "We can only hope that it actually is myocarditis, the acute condition I told you about, which would be connected to this present virus he has. In that case the cough syrup I gave him should gradually get rid of the mucus in his chest, and with rest, as the virus subsides, his heart should begin to get smaller. If it doesn't, we'll have to give a diagnosis of cardiomyopathy, which is a chronic disease of the heart muscle. There is no cure for cardiomyopathy, and Sam will simply have to learn to live with a badly damaged heart. The important thing now is that he do absolutely nothing that could strain it."

"No team sports then?" Parker asked.

"No sports at all. No tennis, no running, no weight lifting, no basketball. He shouldn't even go upstairs quickly."

"What about swimming?" Parker asked, and suddenly

the newspaper picture of Dr. Philip Blaiberg, Christiaan Barnard's successful heart transplant, swimming three months after surgery, flashed into my mind. Swimming was surely good for everyone, and Kent had a brand-new indoor pool.

Oh, good for you, Pa, I thought, but, "No," Tom said flatly. "Oh, he could just paddle around, but no swimming."

"But for how long?" I asked. "He's only seventeen. He'll die if he can't do anything."

Dr. Mansfield politely ignored the obvious corollary. "It's not a question of whether he can climb the Matterhorn this year," he said. "He can't. It's a question of whether he'll be able to do it two years from now. Until we have definite proof that the size of his heart is improving, he simply can't do anything."

I heard Parker saying, "Well, it's okay then if he drives back to Kent tomorrow?"

And Tom answering, "Oh, sure, but tell him if he gets a flat tire to have someone else change it."

The picture of Sam, old Number 71, flagging down a passing car on the turnpike for assistance was even more ludicrous than the one of him paddling in a swimming pool while everyone else jumped, dove, and cannonballed around him.

My God, I thought to myself while Parker and Tom organized the next appointment with Dr. Hall. If it sounds unlikely to me, what the hell will it sound like to Sam?

But there was no arguing with what Tom said. The important thing, Parker and I decided on the way home, was to make Sam understand that he had to play by the rules if he wanted to keep his heart from being permanently damaged. Neither of us wasted a moment considering that it already might be, or that he could have cardiomyopathy, whatever Tom had said that was.

When we got home the troops were assembled as always in the kitchen, exchanging the news of the day. If the Pooles lived in Buckingham Palace, 6 P.M. would still find them tripping all over each other in the palace kitchens. Parker and Sam and I retreated for sanity's sake to the living room in the front of the house and went over the rules.

"But I don't feel sick," he protested once. "How can I be so sick that I can't do anything, if I don't feel bad?"

"You don't want to do something dumb and get knocked out of sports for good, Sam," Parker said. "That damn cough is what you've got to get over so your heart can go back to normal. I know it's rough, but if keeping quiet's going to help, keep quiet."

Walking back to the kitchen, I said, "You'd better enjoy being unaverage, Sam. In two weeks when they do the next echo, your heart probably won't be exciting at all," and he greeted Alix in the kitchen with sadistic pleasure.

"Hard luck, Al. I'm sick, and from now on you have to wait on me. Go get my sneakers out of my room right now. Quick!" and to the assembled multitudes he declared, "See, you guys, I always told you I wasn't an average Joe."

"Yeah, Joe," Pokie admitted with resignation, "Uncle Bill said to tell you he always knew you were a bighearted fellow."

Sam departed for Kent the next morning, and when he came home on January 22 for his next doctor's appointment, he looked like a different person. He was still coughing, but the gray tired look had vanished.

So it was incomprehensible to me the next afternoon when Dr. Hall said, "I'm sorry. It isn't any better. Everything is just the same. With the improvement of the cold he had at Christmas, his heart should be showing improvement too, and it isn't."

If Dr. Mansfield's office was unpretentious, Dr. Hall's was austere. Sam and I sat on two chairs, facing his orderly and uncluttered desk.

"But look at him," I protested. "He looks so much better, and his cold isn't gone by a long shot. He's still coughing."

Dr. Hall was noncommittal. If Sam looked better, it could be attributed to rest. The cough? He shrugged and asked Sam a question or two about the cough medicine Tom Mansfield had prescribed.

He was not noncommittal about what Sam was to do. He was to do nothing. Having added "no drinking" to "no smoking," he startled us both by saying "Fine" to Sam's request to look at colleges over spring vacation.

"I'll look at him again after the trip at the end of March. If there's going to be any improvement, we should see some by then."

"I think you should have told him who you were going on the trip with," I said in the car going home. "I'm sure he thought Daddy and I would be taking you."

What Sam had in mind, I wasn't sure, but it certainly didn't include us. He wanted to go south with three friends from Kent, and it was my guess that colleges would be viewed swiftly while fraternity houses filled with Kent alumni were examined at length. I didn't press the issue. He's had enough nos for one day, I thought, and the letter he wrote us when he got back to Kent the next day made me glad I hadn't. He thanked us for the new camera we gave him as a substitute for his beloved sports and then said:

I did not write before this weekend because I guess I wanted to see what was going to happen to my heart. Now that I know, I feel a lot better because there are no questions as to what I can do. I'll make the best of it. But what has made the biggest difference is knowing I have the best parents behind me. I think I am one of the luckiest people in the world, so thank you for everything.

> I love you both,
> *Sam*

He was a man, and Parker and I had to allow him the dignity of being one, but I felt as if the three of us were adrift in a leaky, unskippered boat.

It was terror that we would sink for lack of bailing that made me call my cousin, H. William Scott, Jr., Professor and Chairman of the Department of Surgery at Vanderbilt University in Nashville. Bill had worked under Dr. Robert Gross, a pioneer in heart surgery at Children's Hospital in Boston, and later under Dr. Alfred Blalock at Johns Hopkins, when the "blue baby" operation was developed. Even Parker, who normally complains about "too many chiefs and not enough Indians," thought it was a good idea.

"Are we doing all we can?" I asked Bill Scott.

"I'll find out," he said.

I gave him Dr. Hall's name and address, and he said that he would ask to have Sam's test results and X-rays sent to Vanderbilt for an appraisal by the cardiology department there.

There was nothing more to do but wait till the end of March for the next echogram. I tried to pretend it was a normal January, with only a few last loads of wash to do for the college troops before they finally returned to the halls of academe, and with only a week for us weary parents to wait before our annual winter escape to St. Kitts in the Leeward Islands.

The day before we were to leave, Parker's mother died, the children all came home again, and, instead of lying on a balmy tropical beach, we found ourselves standing in a New England blizzard beside an open grave in the Poole family plot.

It had been warm and drizzly in the morning, the kind of day that makes you say, "I guess we're going to have the January thaw after all," and we set off for the church in light raincoats. But the temperature plummeted during the service, we arrived in sleet at the cemetery, and by the time poor dear Mrs. Poole was properly interred it was snowing wildly.

It was a macabre scene. The vestments of the Congregational clergyman, who always reminded me of Ichabod Crane, flapped and billowed in the howling wind, and the rest of us huddled together, shivering, at the foot of the grave. I could hear Sam coughing, and I looked down the row of mourners to see him standing, his blond hair covered with snow, with only a bedraggled tweed sports coat to shield him from the wind.

I thought nothing of it when Unkie said, as we walked back to our cars, "Well, I guess that's almost our last trip to this cemetery. There's only room for one more," until Parker added, "I only hope we never have to use it." I knew he'd heard Sam coughing too, and a shudder ran down my spine.

That night we flew to New York and boarded a plane at Kennedy at midnight for our belated vacation. Three hours later we were still on the ground because the baggage-loading equipment was frozen solid.

"We're sorry for the delay, ladies and gentlemen," the disembodied voice of our captain announced, "but occasionally things do foul up."

Parker and I looked at each other and, for the first time since January 5, burst into absolute gales of laughter.

"They do?" I asked him when I could finally control myself.

"Occasionally," he responded, trying to look solemn.

Our vacation was followed by Alix's midwinter vacation, and two days later Charlie and Tina reappeared from Trinity for a ten-day "reading period." I'm convinced that the only thing at private institutions of learning that has out-escalated expenses is vacations. I know for a fact that with a child in private day school, one or two at boarding school, and a couple more at college, it is entirely possible to have someone on vacation nonstop from mid-December until the next year's classes begin in September. To prove the point, Sam appeared on March 13, the day after the Trinityites departed, for his spring vacation.

He looked wonderful. Not since his days of Little League baseball, when, pink-cheeked and rotund, he wedged himself into his Knights of Columbus uniform to attack the forces of the Kippy Cleaners, had he looked so healthy.

"Can you have all this stuff washed for me by tomorrow so I can pack for my trip?" he asked me as he heaved two bursting bags of laundry down the cellar stairs. "Does Dad know I'm leaving Monday? Did Tina leave me Granny's car?"

"Yes, yes, and yes!" I said. I was so delighted with his looks that I would have agreed to wash the laundry for the entire Kent School — and iron it too. "Oh, Sam, you look great."

"I feel great," he said. "I've never felt so well after exams before, even though I'm coughing up a lot more stuff. It's thick, heavy stuff too, but it doesn't tire me out the way it used to, and anyway the rays will fix that."

44

"Rays?" I asked. "What rays? I thought you were going to look at colleges."

"We are, we are, but after I did so well on my exams and all, and after we look at the colleges, don't you think we ought to grab a little Florida sunshine? Think how good it will be for my cough, Mum, and think how great I'll look with a tan."

Parker, who detests cold weather, promptly agreed with him when he got home, and Sam duly departed on Monday morning. He was going to pick up his traveling companions en route, and I'm sure their mothers were assured, as I was, that they wouldn't go near a Florida beach until they'd looked at Gettysburg College, the University of Virginia, Duke, and Chapel Hill.

The Friday after he left, Moriah and I returned to the house from our afternoon walk to find the kitchen electric with moods. Parker had just come home; his was disbelieving. Pokie was just hanging up the telephone; his was amused. Dottie (who had blessedly returned to us in late January) was stirring a chowder at the stove. One look at her back told me that hers was disapproving.

"If he didn't have a bad heart when he went on this trip, he'll certainly have one when he gets back. You mark my words," she declared, turning from the chowder to confront me, the stirring spoon accenting each syllable of her displeasure.

"Aw, come on, Dot," Pokie protested. "He's having a ball. You're only young once."

The spoon was fiercely directed away from me to Pokie. "You certainly didn't need to give him the name of another bar to go to, Parker Poole the Third. I think he's already been in every one from Maine to Florida, and a place called The Wreck, with fifty-cent drinks, that boy doesn't need."

"Florida?" I gasped. "It's only Friday. What about the colleges?"

"Oh, he saw them," Pokie said. "It's just that he can't seem to remember what he saw. He and the other guys spent last night in a parking lot in Cocoa Beach, so he was a little groggy."

"Oh, God," I said to Parker. "What will Dr. Hall say?"

"Don't worry, Mother," Pokie said, obviously thrilled with his protégé. Wedged in between two rather straight-arrow brothers himself, it had been his appointed mission to see that Sam got a taste of the seamy side of life, and Sam delighted in every mouthful. "They have a room in a nice old-ladies' hotel tonight — five dollars a day with a bed, a sink, and four walls. The only trouble is there's only one bed, and the four of them have picked up three other guys."

Granny's car and Sam arrived home together on Wednesday, March 24. Both had aged. Sam's eyes looked like two poached eggs in a bucket of blood.

"Oh, Mum," he groaned, collapsing on one of the ancient Chinese chairs in the front hall and threatening its future. "What a trip! I couldn't be sick. If I really had a bad heart, I'd be dead now."

Two days later, we drove together in my old orange Volkswagen to the hospital for the next echogram. It was a gray and dreary day as only March in Maine can produce, but the weather was no more dismal than I felt.

"Your heart is probably pickled in alcohol after that trip, Sam," I complained. "I expect Dr. Hall will be very grumpy."

"I don't care," he said. "I never even thought about my heart on the trip, and the time I had down there I wouldn't trade for anything. I've got to live my life the way I want to." He swung the car expertly, but much too swiftly, into a slot at the hospital and started off ahead of me through the slush and muck of the parking lot.

After the tests and the echo, we met again in Dr. Hall's office. Dr. Hall handed me a letter and sat at his desk, watching me while I opened it.

It was from Bill Scott, my cousin at Vanderbilt, and I read it eagerly until I came to the second paragraph. The first had been a routine acknowledgment of his receipt of Sam's records, and then I read:

"I have had our chief cardiologist go over the X-rays and echograms, and he entirely concurs with you in your diagnosis of Sam's strange and terrible cardiomyopathy."

The rest of the letter was a blur. I tried to read it, but Sam was looking at me and the words "strange and terrible cardiomyopathy" leapt out at me every time I looked down at the letter.

Oh, dear God, I thought frantically, what if Sam asks to see it? and I folded it up and handed it back to Dr. Hall before he could.

"What'd he say?" Sam asked me, but I just sat there. My throat was so full and tight I couldn't speak. I nodded at Dr. Hall.

"Sam," he said, "it's just what I suspected. Things have not improved. The fact that you've been feeling better is only because you haven't been straining yourself. Your heart is just as enlarged as it was when we took the first X-rays, and there's no hope that it ever will be better. The only thing we can do now is to try to keep it from getting worse. That means sports are out for you for good. I don't plan to give you any medicine right now. In time we'll probably have to start you on digitalis or something along that order, but for now your medicine is keeping just as

47

quiet as you possibly can. I guess that's all there is to say."

Dr. Hall never used the word "cardiomyopathy" and, sitting there, I couldn't remember what Tom Mansfield had said it was except incurable. I couldn't bear to ask in front of Sam.

"Could we have someone else look at him to get an outside opinion?" I asked, forcing my voice to get out the words calmly. It didn't sound like my voice at all. "Would there be any use in it?"

"Oh, absolutely. Of course there's no rush. I don't think things are going to change quickly. But," he added, "I wouldn't get my hopes up that anyone will ever find out what caused the condition. It could have been the mononucleosis he had when he was three, or a strep throat somewhere along the line. It could have been almost anything."

I looked at Sam to see if he had anything to ask. He sat tight-lipped and silent in his chair. His hands were gripping his knees.

I got up to go, and as I did Dr. Hall said to me, "It would be easier for him if he had more intellectual interests, wouldn't it? This must be pretty hard for someone like Sam."

I couldn't answer. "When would you like to see him again?" I asked.

"Well, there's really not much need to keep checking him this regularly now that we know what his problem is. Maybe sometime in May."

Sam and I didn't speak on the way to the Volkswagen. It was parked facing the parking-lot fence. He got in on the driver's side, and I sat beside him. He put both hands on the wheel and slumped forward. Swallowing hard and biting my lip, I stared straight ahead. A sign on the fence said that it was CYCLONE FE. The remains of a snowball covered the NCE. I kept reading the letters over and over, trying to block out the words that were running through my mind: All the king's horses and all the king's men . . . All the king's horses and all the king's men . . .

"Mum," he finally said, and I turned to look at him. Tears were running down his cheeks, and his hands were white-knuckled on the wheel. "Mum, I'm not going to be a damned vegetable."

My self-control broke. Between sobs I cried, "Of course you're not. Oh, darling, of course you're not. Daddy and I will take you anywhere. We'll find the very best heart man in the world, and we'll take you to him. We'll start tonight, and we won't stop until we find someone."

But "all the king's horses and all the king's men" wouldn't stop drumming in my head. What if we go everywhere and there still isn't anything to do? I cried to myself. Don't let me promise what I can't give. Oh, God, don't let Sam be Humpty-Dumpty. Please, God, don't let him be.

I tried to smile between my sniffs, and I put my hand on his shoulder. "I love you," I said, "and Daddy loves you, and the three of us will find someone or something. We won't ever stop, I love you so." I found a wrinkled old Kleenex in my pocketbook and gave him half. "See," I said, "we're all in this together."

Chapter Three

That afternoon in the Volkswagen was high drama for the normally phlegmatic Pooles, but then things reverted to normal. I'd promised Sam that Parker and I would take him anywhere and that we'd fine someone to help him, but in the end "anywhere" turned out to be only Boston, two hours away, and "someone" became a doctor who had been born and brought up in Portland. The whole thing was quite unglamorous, but it took us all of April and most of May even to get that far — two months, one day, and as many sleepless nights since the diagnosis in March of Sam's "strange and terrible cardiomyopathy."

March 26 had seen the end of so many things. For poor old Sam that was the day that dreams of glory faded.

"I guess I'll never row at Henley, Dad," he said to Parker at dinner that night, and there was nothing we could think of to say to make him feel better. He and Charlie had spent the past year sporadically training themselves and continually urging the rest of us to come to England the coming July and watch them sweep to victory. We hadn't mentioned the trip since Sam got sick, and we never did again, but I could have wept for him.

He called us from Kent the night he went back to school after seeing Dr. Hall. "I've told Mr. Perry," he said in a dull, flat voice I'd never heard before. "I've told everybody it's permanent. I can't row anymore."

I thought of the football letter I'd been so uninterested in, and as I hung up I wailed at poor Pokie, my only available audience in the kitchen, "Oh, it just isn't fair."

"Sam will be all right, Mother," Pokie said quietly. "I couldn't do what I wanted either and I survived."

He was perfectly correct. He had survived, and all the years when dreams of glory and varsity letters really count and were impossible for him had long since passed. He could do far more now with a hand and a half than I could with two, but it didn't take the sting away that night.

"But don't you see, Pokie," I protested angrily, "it wasn't fair for you either," and I refused to listen to Mother's voice asking a petulant fourteen-year-old me, "Vicky, who ever told you life was fair?"

What ended for me on March 26 was sleep, and I did a pretty good job of ending it for Parker too. He had given me a digital clock for Christmas, and the night after I read Bill Scott's letter the digits and I became intimately acquainted.

At 2:07 that night I woke up. At 2:31 I tried to recite poetry, but for some strange reason the only poem I could muster was Emily Dickinson's "I Heard a Fly Buzz When I Died," and I couldn't even dredge up the second line. At 3:29 I woke up Parker.

"I hate this clock," I said. "I will know precisely when I die, and I don't want to."

"Unplug it," he groaned.

"I don't want to," I said. "I want to talk about Sam. We've got to take him somewhere."

"I know. I've already decided to call Dr. Hall in the morning. Now go to sleep."

Worry filled every day and every night. Infinite and uninvited, it intruded upon our lives, and even the seemingly simple task of getting an outside opinion on Sam became fraught with anxiety. Dr. Hall made an appointment for him with a cardiologist at Peter Bent Brigham Hospital in Boston, but no one seemed to know who had recommended him or what his qualifications were.

It wasn't until the end of April that something finally went right, and it only came about because of a shameless extravagance that Parker and I make almost annually. Parker likes St. Kitts best in January when he's cold but, as I hate going home to face winter again, I prefer St. Kitts in April. So we go both times. Our self-indulgence paid off that spring. Georgie Bowers, who with her husband Bill owns and runs the hotel where we stay, was aghast at what had happened to us just since February. And she knew a doctor who used to be head of cardiology at the Massachusetts General Hospital.

"He was so important," she said, "that he was the one who decided who was eligible to be sent off for a heart transplant and who wasn't. Not that Sam's that badly off, but it never hurts to go to the top," and she fired off a letter to him about Sam that night.

"At least," she said comfortingly, "you can call him when you get home, and he can tell you if the doctor Sam has the appointment with is okay."

The former head of cardiology at Mass General had never heard of the man at Peter Bent Brigham, his secretary informed me when I called his office the day after we got back to Maine, and that was too much for Parker. He called Dr. Hall. "I told him that we want Sam to see someone who is absolutely the best in his field," he reported back to me.

The Peter Bent Brigham appointment was canceled. Dr. Hall set up an appointment with Dr. J. Alfred Owens, Assistant Professor of Medicine at Mass General, and this time the former head of cardiology assured me we were in good hands. I could only wonder why Dr. Hall hadn't produced Dr. Owens in the first place. Not only did Dr. Owens's Portland origins make him an obvious choice, but he was a friend of Tom Mansfield's to boot.

Nothing made any sense anymore, and, other than Georgie Bowers's medical connections, it was hard to find anything to recommend getting up in the morning to face another day. The only bright spot on the whole gloomy horizon was the upcoming sale of my parents' winter house. Someone had finally agreed with Daddy's opinion of it and put down what Parker called "earnest money."

My mirror regularly and unkindly informed me that no one over forty should worry and that whatever Dr. Erno Laszlo's gold-plated face potions were supposed to be combating, they weren't. Worst of all, my social graces were deteriorating. In a fearsomely chic New York restaurant with Rozzie and Ruth and Malcolm earlier in the month, I had fallen asleep sitting bolt upright eating my dinner, which was bad enough, but when I woke up asking "What size tennis dress does Charlie wear?" even Rozzie, who was getting used to the new me, shook her head with dismay.

On Thursday, May 27, Parker and I drove to Boston to meet Sam at Mass General and see Dr. Owens. Charlie had picked up Sam up at Kent on Wednesday afternoon, bedded him down at Trinity for the night, and was under Parker's explicit orders to "Get him out of bed in time to be in Boston at quarter of eleven and tell him we'll meet him at the main entrance of the hospital. I don't *care* what he's like in the morning, Charles. You just get him up!"

It was spring as spring should be — and rarely is in Maine — that morning, but I looked at the green grass and the apple blossoms with a jaundiced eye as we drove along. It was plain that my misery had company in Parker. He looked so tired as we drove into the hospital parking lot that I forced myself to make a bedraggled attempt at optimism. I gave him a pat and said, "Well, maybe today we'll find out that things aren't as bad as we thought."

"If we find Sam, we'll be doing well," he answered, eyeing the massive brick-and-concrete complex spread out before us, and I was inclined to agree with him as we walked inside.

There seemed to be some question in the minds of the staff, as well as in ours, as to what actually constituted the main entrance of the hospital, so Parker positioned himself in one possible area while I waited in another. To my complete amazement Sam walked through the glass entry doors of my section at precisely ten forty-five.

The first thing I thought was that if I'd been a lumpy seventeen-year-old again and no relative, he would never have wasted a minute on me. He was so handsome he made me feel nervous, and his tan, courtesy of the Florida rays, was outrageously becoming. His sun-bleached hair curled properly over the collar of his properly faded blue shirt, which was tucked into a pair of properly rumpled corduroys. On his feet his Adidas were more properly scruffy than ever, and I dared give him no more than a properly motherly kiss before we set off to find Parker.

Sam said Charlie hadn't let him take time to eat break-fast, and I had my next thought about him when the three of us were sitting in the coffee shop. He was strangely sub-dued, and the toneless voice I'd first noticed over the tele-phone after he went back to Kent seemed to have become his normal way of speaking. What he said came out mostly in monosyllables, few, far between, and delivered with effort.

How did he feel? "Fine." How was the cough? "Still there. I got another cold last week."

He did tell us, though, that he'd been "tapped" on Mon-day night and had kept it as a surprise for us for today. Tapping at Kent is a big thing, because it is the way the top ten school leaders for the final sixth-form year are an-nounced. Not only does it bestow all kinds of eminence upon the recipient of the tap, but it also doesn't hurt a bit as far as getting into college is concerned. Poole academics being what they are, it was an acknowledged blessing that Parker's genes for leadership and not mine were trans-ferred to the next generation. (My one term of office as class president was served in the last half of the second grade.)

At any rate, Sam was going to be the head of Blue Key, thereby responsible for hospitality and entertainment at Kent. He was thoroughly relieved not to find himself a pre-fect, as Malcolm and Charlie had been — "God, Mum, that would have been awful. I've got enough trouble keeping my own nose clean without worrying about anybody else's" — and also relieved at not being made a verger and in charge of the chapel like Tina — "God, Mum, religion's not my thing!"

"You're right," I said, as we made our way through a maze of subterranean passages to find Dr. Owens's office. "Blue Key will be a perfect job for you. If you can't do sports, at least you'll be so busy organizing everybody's social life you won't have time to miss them."

"Oh, I'm doing sports," he said. "I started playing tennis when I went back after vacation. I told you I won't be a vegetable."

I stopped dead in my tracks. "What do you mean?" I said. "Dr. Hall said you shouldn't do anything!"

"Come on, come on," Parker interrupted. "Don't argue about it here. We'll be late. It doesn't seem to be killing him, and we can ask Dr. Owens about it after he's looked at him."

Sam was sent off, with us trailing along behind, for an electrocardiogram — an EKG, in hospitalese — and a chest X-ray before we saw Dr. Owens. When we returned to the narrow hall which served as his waiting room, we sat down on an even narrower bench next to a vigorously Boston lady and her frail daughter. At one point, when her mother rose off the bench with some impatience, the wan girl feebly raised the thinnest arm I had ever seen, as if to pull her back.

I couldn't keep myself from staring. I had always carried a picture in my mind of T. S. Eliot's Princess Volupine extending her "meagre, blue-nailed, phthisic hand" because I loved the "phthisic," but suddenly there was the hand itself attached to a child no older than Sam. I tore my eyes away from the girl to look at him. A very brown, very large hand rested on his knee, and the nails comfortingly belonged to any seventeen-year-old boy whose nail brush had got lost the first week of school. Even so, I was shamelessly glad to leave the girl and her mother behind when we were called into Dr. Owens's office.

I've never quite decided whether it was the vast amount of Maine memorabilia that Dr. Owens had brought with him or his easy manner that made Sam feel at home. In less than two minutes, though, the taciturn patient of Dr. Hall's office had vanished along with the morning's monosyllables, and, while Parker and I listened disbelievingly, he told Dr. Owens exactly what he'd been doing since he decided not to be a vegetable. Tennis, basketball, swimming, and "I still run upstairs. God, I'd never get to class if I didn't."

It didn't seem to disturb Dr. Owens at all. He was examining Sam, inspecting his ankles closely — "for signs of edema," he explained; "when fluid is retained, the ankles are the first place to show swelling" — poking and prodding his stomach, and listening to his heart. From time to time he would pause to quiz us on symptoms, family history, physical injuries. I had emptied our family closet of its only medically related skeleton, my grandfather, A. R. Wright, who had died of a heart attack at fifty-three, and I had run through Sam's age-three bout with mono. Parker had brought up a forgotten injury that Sam had suffered the previous November, when he fell on top of a football and tore the rib cartilage on the left side of his chest.

Our well of disorders had almost run dry when Sam suddenly announced: "I passed out the other day at school. It must have been flu or something, but when I stood up I felt all dizzy and fell down."

Parker and I looked at him sharply. "You didn't tell us that," Parker said.

"I guess I didn't" was the reply, and it didn't occur to either of us to bring up the time at Sugarloaf when he had almost passed out skiing.

After he finished looking at Sam, Dr. Owens sat on the edge of his desk and gave us his opinion. Sam was assuredly suffering from some as yet undetermined form of cardiomyopathy, but "except for his heart," he said with enthusiasm, "he's in wonderful physical shape."

That seemed to bear all the melancholy overtones of "And aside from that, Mrs. Lincoln, did you enjoy the play?" but I sat there, trying to listen with a positive attitude, while he went on to list the things that he had observed about Sam's condition. His cardiogram was normal. The X-ray he'd had in the morning and the results of previous echoes indicated that his valves and arteries were perfectly all right, but, listening to Sam's heart, he had detected a third sound, a gallop, which ought not to be there. He also said that Sam should start taking aspirin four times a day to forestall blood clots. With a heart as badly enlarged as his was, the pumping action of the heart muscle was very weak, the heart chambers were not properly flushed, and the blood left behind grew sludgy.

On a piece of yellow legal paper, he drew us a picture of Sam's heart. It was oddly misshapen, with an obscene bulge on the left side, and the three of us peered intently at the paper while he drew a dotted line inside. It followed far more closely the contours of hearts as I remembered them from my days in Biology I.

"The dotted line shows what would be happening to Sam's heart if the enlargement had been caused by a temporary condition. If the heart muscle hadn't suffered permanent damage, the heart itself would be getting smaller, and we could say that he had myocarditis," he explained, writing the word next to the heart.

He pointed then to the outer lines of his drawing. "With cardiomyopathy, the heart muscle has been irrevocably damaged, and nothing can be done to reduce the enlargement of the heart," he said. "We can only try to keep it from getting worse."

Under "myocarditis" he wrote "cardiomyopathy," and, for the first time I saw printed out together the two words that had by now become part of Poole household vernacular. For the first time too, thanks to Dr. Owens's drawing, I could finally see exactly what Sam's problem was, and I could — if I'd felt like it, but I didn't — take some smug satisfaction in Dr. Owens's determination that Sam should have a heart catheterization done when he got out of school in June. It could be done in our local hospital.

"It would be three months before we could schedule him here," he said, "and they can do it just as well in Portland."

In my pocketbook I had a list of things we wanted to ask, carefully compiled during our 3 A.M. conferences, but, just as I was about to reach for it, Dr. Owens's telephone rang and ended our appointment. He had an emergency, he explained, as he rushed out the door. He would write Dr. Hall and Tom Mansfield.

The entire appointment we'd waited for and worried about for so long had lasted twenty minutes from start to finish, and, although we all concluded that it had been very worthwhile, we didn't quite know why. We were still in a daze of unasked questions and bewildered silence after lunch as we watched Sam set off for Kent.

"Be sure to pick up some aspirin," we yelled at him as he drove off in the old blue Volvo station wagon which was yet another symbol of the frustrations that had dogged our footsteps since March 26. We had bought it for him during spring vacation, hoping to ensure his mobility to and from doctor's appointments since there's no way to get to Kent from Maine by means of public transportation. Kent, however, with good reason forbade student vehicles, and Hart Perry had sounded so dubious about a car for medical purposes that it had to be garaged at Trinity, more than an hour away. Every time we needed Sam, Charlie or Tina had to make a cross-country pilgrimage to get him to his wheels.

"His car will probably break down on the way back to Trinity, and he'll forget all about getting the aspirin," I groaned, as Parker and I started off for home. "Do you realize that we never had a chance to ask Dr. Owens what he thought about the things Sam was doing, and he never said a word when Sam told him. What do we do now?"

We were still asking ourselves that question when we got back to Portland about four thirty, and we still had no answer. I felt disagreeably incomplete.

"I can't bear to go back to that damn mausoleum," I said. "Let's go out to the Cape and look at the house."

The Cape is the name we use to distinguish the family land — bought by my grandmother in 1913 — from the town of Cape Elizabeth, in which it is situated. My parents' summer house (which was still far from ready for the wall-papers rushed from New York by the interior decorators) is there, and within easy strolling distance on the property are Bill and Rozzie's summer cottage and ours, as well as our cousins' summer houses. Selling the winter house in town was only selling memories, but to sell the Cape would have been to sell our souls. Every tree, every field, and every inch of that land is dearly beloved by us all.

We drove in the back driveway by the pond, and everything was so green and so beautiful that it seemed almost indecent to have troubles. Rozzie was in her usual bent-double position in her garden, and she gave us a cheerful upside-down wave as we drove by.

In the fall before Sam got sick, we had decided to add on a new living room and bedroom to the house, trustingly presuming that the existing building would need little more than fresh paint and paper to make it perfect. We were wrong, and, when I saw that the contractor's truck was still there that afternoon, I let Parker go into the house alone to check on the day's progress. I didn't have the fortitude to hear what sinister new symptom of rot and decay had been unearthed since the day before, and I started down the path toward the garden to find Rozzie.

She was just coming up to the house, and we met outside the kitchen at the old stone wall that separates lawn from woods. To my horror and for no accountable reason, I took one look at her and burst into tears.

"What is it?" she kept saying, but I only stood there sobbing and shaking my head.

Rozzie is rarely demonstrative, but she flung both her arms around me and sat me down on the wall beside her, hugging me as if I were ten years old again. "You and Uncle Parker come right home with me," she said. "What you need is a nice drink with Uncle Billy."

She is always perceptive, and her prescription returned me to my more stolid self. When we got home I put the yellow paper Dr. Owens had given us on the bulletin board in the kitchen and began the study of Sam's heart and of the word "cardiomyopathy" that became a daily occupation.

We got a copy of Dr. Owens's letter to Dr. Hall a week later, on June 4. He mentioned a slight ("subtle," he called it) change for the worse in the heart's size since the January X-rays. He also described the gallop sound he had detected and recommended that cardiac catheterization be done "to establish at this point in time what the nature of his heart disease is and what limitations if any should be imposed."

He said again that Sam was in excellent physical condition, which again served only to depress me. "God, it's as bad as saying, 'The operation was a success, but the patient died,' " I said bitterly to Parker as he read the letter.

Dr. Hall arranged to have the catheterization done by Dr. Philip Wakely, a cardiologist at our Portland hospital, on June 21. Sam would be admitted to the hospital on the twentieth and released on the twenty-second, the first anniversary of Daddy's death.

Sam came home from Kent on June 14 after a detour to two end-of-school bashes and spent most of the week helping me move to the cottage at the Cape. When work started on my parents' summer house, we had asked the contractor to promise that it would be completely habitable by June. He had given his vow, but we knew — and we knew he knew — that we'd be lucky to move in before snow flew. We had never doubted for a moment that the cottage on the beach, five hundred feet down the field, would be Poole headquarters for yet another season, and everyone was delighted to get back to its rambling and ramshackle simplicity after our winter of enforced splendor.

We had our first picnic of the summer season at Bill and Rozzie's swimming pool, halfway between their summer cottage and ours, on the Sunday Sam went to the hospital for his catheterization. He and I left about two. He was very quiet, as he'd been since he came home. I'd begun to wonder if I had imagined the bedlam which used to emanate from the big room he shared with Charlie behind the kitchen, and I would have given my eyeteeth to have a raucous rendition of "The Wild Weed Flower" and the perils of growing marijuana assault my ear. There hadn't been any foolishness at all since he came home.

It was miserably hot in Portland that afternoon, and the hospital was the last place anyone would choose to be. Sam was admitted and put in a semiprivate room, where he was duly attended by one of Dr. Wakely's associates.

Oddly enough, I wasn't nervous at all about the catheterization, and Sam certainly didn't act as though he were. Three days before, he and Parker and I had met with Dr. Wakely in his office to have the process explained and the potential risks outlined. I had come away with the impression that a catheterization was unpleasant, but not unendurable, and that the risks involved for Sam were more or less routine. They sounded like standard "having your wisdom teeth out" ones, except of course for the consideration of Sam's heart condition, which created some slight additional concern. I had definitely come away liking Dr. Wakely.

To Parker's continual dismay, and in most un-Maine-ish manner, I decide with one glance if I'm going to hate someone. It usually takes me much longer to decide about someone I might like, but not with Dr. Wakely. He was small and dark, with the kindest eyes I have ever seen, and he had seemed to like Sam. That was enough for me, but I must have been concentrating so hard on him that I didn't completely grasp all the things he told us. Rozzie complained, when we got home and I tried to explain them to her, that I made no sense at all. I was very grateful to hear Dr. Wakely's associate describe a cardiac catheterization all over again in Sam's hospital room.

A small incision would be made in Sam's forearm and a thin tube, or catheter, snaked through a vein into the right side of the heart. Pressure would be recorded at rest and during exercise, as Dr. Owens wanted to test Sam's heart under strain. Once this portion of the test was completed, a second catheter would be introduced into an artery through a small puncture in the right groin. From there it would be advanced through to the aorta, the main artery leading from the heart, and into the left ventricle, the main left pumping chamber. At that point a radio contrast liquid (when I said, "A what?" he said, "Well, I expect you'd understand it better if I called it a dye, but that wouldn't be correct") would be released into the left ventricle during a motion-picture X-ray to determine the strength of the heart's contractions.

It sounded quite reasonable, and after he departed a resident interviewed Sam, an intern reinterviewed him, and a pretty young nurse cut off the legs of the hospital pajamas she had issued him.

"It's too hot to have anything on," she said.

The catheterization was to take place at nine the next morning, but when I got to the hospital at eight thirty to give Sam a motherly sendoff, he had disappeared. They had taken him up to the Cardiology Department at eight, and eleven thirty would be, they thought, a realistic time for me to check in there.

At eleven fifteen Parker and I were accordingly sitting on the sofa in the large hallway that comprised the waiting room of Cardiology. We had spent so many hours there waiting for echos and EKGs to be done that we should have felt at home, but we looked nervously at every door that opened or closed for fear we might miss Dr. Wakely.

We could have relaxed, because we were obviously very much on Dr. Wakely's mind as he came out of the area where the catheterizations were done. "Oh, there you are," he cried as he spotted us. "I was hoping you'd be here. I'm sorry it took so long, but the bicycle we were using for the exercise part of the study kept breaking down. Poor old Sam's had an awfully rough morning."

My snap judgment of Dr. Wakely had been absolutely

correct. He did really seem to care about Sam. He smiled then and said, "You know, I forgot to tell you at the office the other day that I was one of the first people to see the chest X-rays he had taken in January. I just happened to be hanging around the X-ray Department when the radiologists were studying his films, and they asked my opinion. When I saw them I couldn't believe my eyes. I only wish it hadn't had to be Sam, but if it had to be, I'm glad I could do his catheterization. He should get a medal for what he put up with today."

It seemed that every time Sam had been told to pedal, the bicycle had balked. "He was great, though," Dr. Wakely said. "He even tried to help us fix it. He never complained once, and we've had older people who haven't had to put up with the discomfort of two catheters who've given us all kinds of trouble. He's a sweet kid," he said, just as Sam was wheeled out on a stretcher into the hall.

Dr. Wakely was still in his scrub suit, and he had a clear plastic package in his hand. When he saw Sam he walked over to him and handed him the package.

"Here are the catheters we used on you, Sam. I guess they'll have to do for your medals. They cost seventy dollars, and, wasteful as it is, we can't use them again. Maybe you can think of something to do with them, but anyway I've just been telling your parents what a great job you did this morning. We'd never have gotten that bicycle working without you."

Sam was very much the genial host as he lay on his stretcher. Two nurses were positively beaming down on him with motherly pride, and he started to tease Dr. Wakely about the bicycle.

"I'd hate to have to depend on that for transportation," he said, and Dr. Wakely grinned back at him. It was quite

65

obvious that they had enjoyed each other's company during the morning's activities.

Dr. Wakely departed, with a comradely pat of Sam's shoulder, and Parker and I followed the stretcher and Sam back to his room. For all his good spirits with Dr. Wakely and the nurses, the catheterization had obviously exhausted him. When I asked him if it had hurt, he only said, "Just parts of it," but then, lying on his side in the bed with his eyes closed, he added in a groggy voice, "It wasn't that it was so bad. It's just it took so long and I'm so tired."

He'd had some sedation before the catheterization — not much, Dr. Wakely said, because he had to be alert enough to cope with the bicycle — and he obviously wanted to sleep, so I went back to the house in town to pack up the last of the Poole bits and pieces and to wait for Dr. Wakely to call with the results.

He called about four. I was in the kitchen, and through the open windows came all the sounds of a hot June afternoon. I could hear a lawn mower purring its way across one neighbor's yard and the happy pandemonium of children playing in another's as Dr. Wakely told me that the reports about Sam's heart had not been exaggerated. The tests that had gone before had been inaccurate only in not showing how hideously damaged it was.

I don't remember being surprised or even upset by what he said. For some strange reason it was a relief to finally know the worst, and I found myself asking point-blank the question that had been in my mind since we'd heard that Sam's heart would never get better. Before today I had squelched it with an "Aren't we overdramatizing a bit?" to myself, and the one time I'd mentioned it to Parker, he'd told me not to be ridiculous.

"Dr. Wakely," I said, "will this shorten Sam's life?"

"It will have to," he said almost petulantly, as if he were irritated and impatient with the medical laws that had made him reach such a terrible conclusion.

I don't recall another thing we said after that, but at nine o'clock the next morning, Parker and I were waiting again in Cardiology to talk to him, so I must have arranged the meeting. Sam had seemed so depressed the night after the catheterization that I had made a special effort to look nice that morning. It was bad enough to have heart trouble without having a mother you were embarrassed to be seen with come to take you home, and I had put on a pair of pristine white slacks and a white T-shirt (purchased at a most un-T-shirtish price) with little splashes of bright pink on it.

When Dr. Wakely appeared, he said, "I'd like to show you the film of Sam's heart before we talk. I think it will help you to understand what his problem is."

We followed him into a small room near the section of Cardiology where catheterizations were done. A doctor who was the father of one of Alix's best friends was just leaving the room, and we all smiled and bowed as politely and calmly as though we were at a PTA meeting.

"I'd like you to look at this film of a normal heart before you look at Sam's," Dr. Wakely said, putting a reel on a projector. On a small screen, rather like a portable television set, we saw a heart pumping. It belonged, Dr. Wakely explained, to a healthy forty-year-old woman, and it was in the middle of the screen, doing what a heart ought to do. As the heart walls compressed with the forceful pumping action, the blood could be seen flowing out of the left ventricle into the aorta, leaving the chamber virtually empty.

"Now," he said, "here's Sam's."

Unlike the other film, which had no introduction, Sam's

had credits exactly as though we were about to view "Saturday Night at the Movies." *T. S. Poole* was the title, and it was followed by the date and what Dr. Wakely identified as the catheterization number. The hospital's Cath Lab was the producer. The plot was sickening.

"You can't see the entire heart," Dr. Wakely said. "It's so enlarged, particularly on the left side, that it goes right off the screen."

We could see the contrast liquid coming into the heart, and we could faintly — but only faintly — detect a pumping action. The heart walls would compress ever so slightly, but at the bottom of the heart there was a centrifugally sloshing mass of blood that never left the chamber at all.

"Less than twenty-five percent of the blood leaves his heart when it beats," Dr. Wakely said, and I immediately understood Dr. Owens's concern about blood clots. It required little imagination, having seen the film, to picture the consistency of the blood left behind in Sam's heart. Like cream left over from last week's dinner party, it would grow thicker and sludgier every day.

Parker hadn't said anything the night before when I told him what I'd asked Dr. Wakely except, "Let's wait till tomorrow when we know the whole story." I knew that he hoped I'd been looking on the dark side again and had either overdramatized or at least misinterpreted Dr. Wakely's answer. I wished he'd been right.

"Dr. Wakely," I said, "by how much will this shorten Sam's life?"

It was hard to guess, he said, shaking his head. Sam could live a few more years, maybe even five, if he took it easy. He couldn't possibly live more than ten, regardless of how careful he was, and there was always the chance that he could throw a blood clot at any time. "Or," he finished, "his heart could just give out."

Parker and I didn't say anything. There didn't seem to be anything to say, and in the silence Dr. Wakely must have wondered if we had completely understood him.

He leaned forward in his chair. "This is like telling parents that their child has leukemia," he said, "except that it's worse because there is absolutely no cure. There are all kinds of things they can do now to arrest leukemia, and some types of it can even be cured, but there is not one thing we can do to help Sam. The only thing that could possibly prolong his life would be a heart transplant, and, as I'm sure you know, a heart transplant is no cure. Somewhere down the line, though, you're going to have to consider one."

It seemed so much easier to listen to his words than to consider their ramifications that I remember perfectly what he said. He told us about the rejections that complicate organ transplantation and explained that of course with kidneys the hazards of rejection could be cut down by taking the transplant from a family member. Obviously, with hearts you couldn't hope for such compatibility because —

He stopped right in the middle of his sentence and peered at us intently. "I know you have a big family," he said. "You don't by any possible chance have another child who has an inoperable brain tumor or something?"

It was such a dreadful thought that we were both stunned. I looked questioningly at Parker and he looked questioningly at me, and then we both, almost apologetically, shook our heads.

To this day, Dr. Wakely swears he couldn't have said such a thing. "It would be quite out of character," he says, but both Parker and I clearly remember that he did. It was absolutely plain, though, that the question was prompted only by a desire to help Sam. Dr. Wakely looked quite as miserable and depressed as we did, and the three of us sat there in the little room without speaking after that. I kept looking at the pink splashes on my T-shirt. They were shaped like little teardrops.

Once I looked over at Parker. His expression was as impassive as ever, but I could imagine what was happening to him inside, and I went back to my study of the splashes. To have things beyond his control is unbearable for him; to have things run as they should for his family is his unalterable goal. Protestations of love you don't get from Parker, but twenty times a day that love is revealed by what he does.

Dr. Wakely didn't know either of us, though, and I wonder from time to time what he thought of us that morning. I wonder if he realized that self-control was the only sanity we had left. In our quietness, he might well have thought we were cold-blooded.

In any case he was very gentle. "You got a copy of Dr. Owens's letter to Dr. Hall, didn't you? He mentioned the possibility of a heart transplant in that."

I looked at him blankly. Was I going mad? "We got the letter," I said, "but it didn't say anything about a heart transplant."

"Oh, that's right, Dr. Hall had that part deleted from your copy. Would you like to see it now?" He retrieved Dr. Owens's letter from a manila folder that must have held Sam's file and handed it to me. It was exactly like the one we had received, but it had one more paragraph, about a transplant.

Walking to the elevator to go down to Sam's room, we

met Dr. Hall. Dr. Wakely was with us, and, after Dr. Hall had told us how sorry he was about and for Sam, Dr. Wakely said, "I told them about the possible eventuality of a heart transplant, George."

Dr. Hall looked surprised. "Oh, that's years down the road," he said, brusquely brushing it off. "There's no need to even think about that now."

I had assumed that Dr. Wakely had become Sam's doctor, but Dr. Hall told us to let him know if anything out of the ordinary troubled him, "any numbness in his hands or swelling in his ankles, for example," and told us to keep in touch. "I ought to check him over before he goes back to school in the fall," he said, "but in the meantime he can take a vacation from doctors. I'm sure he won't mind, and I guess that's all there is to say for now. Phil's going down with you to go over things with Sam, isn't he?"

Dr. Wakely nodded, and the three of us got into the elevator and went down to Sam's room. His roommate was in the other bed, so Dr. Wakely trotted down the hall until he found an empty room and beckoned us in behind him. As I remember we were all quite jovial, including Sam, and Parker and I leaned against the broad window ledge while Dr. Wakely and Sam bargained back and forth in the best of humor about the life-style of a cardiac patient.

"But how can I sit in a bar all night and only have one beer? It'll ruin my image!"

"Drink the one beer slowly, Sam."

"You mean I can't unload boxcars this summer? What'll happen to my muscles?"

"You've got plenty of muscle already."

"Well, can I go home now?"

"Sure, but we'll miss you. You're sure you don't want to stick around?"

"No, that's okay, Dr. Wakely. I'll see you later."

I looked at my watch and it was only nine forty-five. Sam was going to die, and it had all taken less than forty-five minutes.

Parker went back to the office, and I waited while Sam pulled on his jeans, put on his Adidas, and stuck his toothbrush in his pocket. That, with the catheters and a book, comprised his luggage.

"Can I take the car and go find Fred?" he asked. "God, I can't wait to get out of this place."

"Sure," I said. "You can drop me off at the cemetery, and I'll go home with Aunt Roz."

I had told Rozzie the night before that she would have to go without me to meet the man from Murphy's Monuments at the cemetery where the family is buried. In May, before Sam's catheterization was set up, we realized with horror that the anniversary of Daddy's death was fast approaching, and he and Mother still had no tombstones. We had picked the anniversary of Daddy's death to order the stones because we knew we would never forget to be there on that day, and both of us were becoming subject to visions of Daddy opening the lid of his coffin to bellow at passersby, "These goddamned girls can't do anything right!"

I must have been in a state of shock or else in perfect control of myself, because Sam and I talked cheerfully all the way to the cemetery about what a great guy Dr. Wakely was, how great it was that the catheterization was over, and how great the summer would be with no more dumb doctors' appointments to worry about.

It wasn't till I got out of the car at the family plot that I began to fall apart. This is grotesque, I thought. What am I doing in this damn place when Sam is going to die?

Rozzie was deeply engrossed with the man from Murphy's Monuments, and it wasn't until Sam yelled, "Hi, Aunt Roz," out of the window of the Volkswagen that she turned around and saw us.

"Oh, Say-am," she cried, using the pronunciation of his name that was the relic of a trip to Wyoming she'd taken him on, and she ran down the banking from the graves toward us. "How did it go?"

"Great," Sam yelled back. "It's all over," and he drove away.

Mr. Murphy's man was precise and interminably long-winded, which I expect, considering the permanence of his product, was understandable, but I heartily detested him. It seemed that we would never succeed in making Mother DOROTHY WRIGHT, BELOVED WIFE OF CHARLES FREDERIC SIMES, and it must have been well after eleven when he finally departed.

"Now, tell me," Rozzie said.

"Oh, Rozzie," I said, "you were right. Only it's worse than leukemia. He's going to die," and I sat down on Daddy's grave and put my head on my knees and wept.

Our sister Louise and our brother John are buried between Mother and Daddy, and Rozzie sat down on Johnnie's grave and wept too. Anyone going by who remembered that Daddy had died exactly twelve months before might well have commented, "Well, the Simes girls haven't gotten very far this year, have they?"

It wasn't until Rozzie looked up and realized that we had become the object of contemplation for a group of lunching gravediggers that she nudged me. There they sat, munching on their sandwiches with their shovels beside them, staring at us in rapt fascination, so we got up and went home.

Chapter Four

Sometime during the twenty-five-minute trip home from the cemetery, Rozzie must have stopped crying because when we got to the cottage she said firmly, "Vicky, I've been talking to Mother, and she says this is not the time to cry. She says there will be plenty of time for that if Sam does die, but for now we've got to help him, and crying won't."

If Rozzie had offered the statement as her own, I wouldn't have listened to her, and my personal opinion on any matter of importance wouldn't have interested her a bit either. But ever since Mother died, we had used her as our common authority, prefixing dicta with, "I just talked to Mother and she says . . ."

"I know," I said. "She's right. Thanks," and I got out of the car and went into the cottage. Dottie was ironing in the little room between the kitchen and Sam and Charlie's bedroom, and I went in to tell her.

Dottie and I have, as she puts it, an unusual employer-employee relationship. Because she is at least three inches taller than I am and considerably more majestic, I rarely emerge from debates with her feeling the victor. With one arched eyebrow, with a single sniff, with one toss of her jet black hair, she conveys more displeasure with a disobedient child or an erring parent than could any two-hour lecture. (I am a lecturer by nature, and I know.)

Her mother, who had sewed for all of us from the time I was thirteen until she died in 1974, had directed her always to address me as "Mrs. Poole." As the years have progessed, and as our friendship has deepened, when she's found the pot I burned from last night's supper or when I come home from a party with a spot on my dress, I am quite as often "Mrs. Poole, you slob," and I would never effect a change in our lives or in the children's lives without first consulting her.

I sat down facing her on the lumpy old cot where we fold the laundry, but I couldn't bring myself to tell her about Sam.

"My Dottie," he used to say when he was little, putting his arms around her ample person.

"My Dottie," one of the older children would tease, running to her and putting their arms around her too.

"There'll be no fighting," Dottie would dictate. "There's enough to go around for everybody." I needed my share that day.

After a minute she looked up from the corduroys she was ironing and said quietly, "Bad news, huh?"

"Awful," I said. "The worst."

"Are you going to tell the other kids?" she asked, going back to her ironing.

I hadn't even thought about that, but I instantly said, "Oh, no. They'd act differently toward him and he'd know somehow. Oh, not yet."

The house was unfamiliarly quiet. Alix was off at a

friend's for the day, Tina and Pokie were working, and that morning Charlie had flown from Hartford to England to train with the Trinity crew for the Henley. It had been hard to say good-bye to him on the phone the night before, with Sam, who would never row again, in the hospital and all the memories of the family trip we'd planned rushing back.

"Tell Sam I'll miss him," Charlie had said. "Tell him I'll try to row for him too."

I trailed along behind Dottie and her chores like one of the children most of the afternoon, and oddly enough it was Sam himself who brought things back to normal. He and a friend, Craig Clark, burst into the kitchen about four, exultantly flourishing large brown paper bags at us. "You're about to view a new million-dollar corporation," Sam announced as Dottie and I stared at the two of them. "Dad's hired us both for the summer. And look!"

From the paper bags came matching dark green work shirts. On the pocket in front, Sam's said *Sam* and Craig's said *Craig*, and on the back of both in large yellow letters was stitched C & P Painting Co.

"Clark and Poole, Mum," he went on. "Get it?"

"Of course I get it, Sam," I said haughtily, delighted that he was in such good spirits. "But do you mean a million dollars in debts or assets? Why do you have to spend money for uniforms just to paint on Dad's wharf?"

He looked pained. "It's image, Mum. Ya gotta have image. Gawd, only an average Joe would paint without a uniform." And shaking his head, he and Craig went out to the back bedroom to try on their new images, leaving Dottie and me behind in the kitchen, impressed with Parker's resourcefulness. Sam and I had parted company at ten that morning and now here he was, cardiomyopathy and all, with a full-fledged summer job.

Working on the W. H. Shurtleff Company wharves in the summer is a symbol of manhood to male Pooles. Like his father and his brothers before him (except for Charlie, who became a lobsterman at ten), Sam had been unloading boxcars since he was fifteen, and I knew that in his mind no other occupation could compete with the camaraderie to be found at the Shurtleff branch of Local 340 of the Teamsters' Union. He had taken Dr. Wakely's orders against boxcar unloading without complaint, but I knew he was dreading a summer without a job, and evidently Parker knew it even better than I did.

That morning at the hospital, Dr. Wakely had okayed painting for Sam, and Parker decided that there was plenty of painting that needed to be done among the twenty-odd sheds and offices on the two wharves. It crossed his mind, too, that Sam would enjoy his job a lot more if he had someone working with him, and it would be safer to have someone else around in case anything went wrong. Bad heart or not, Sam still had to feel a part of things.

"And there's no better place to feel a part of things," Parker told me that night when he came home, "than down on those damned wharves. He can goof off playing penny-ante poker with the guys and be right in his element. That's what he'd really miss anyway."

"Oh, Pa," I said, "there's nobody like you, but where did you find Sam? When he left me off at the cemetery, he said he was going to find Freddie."

I should have known better than to ask. When Sam couldn't find Fred, he went at noon to where everyone else goes at noon when they feel a need to talk to Parker: he went to the tugboat.

It seems almost the last straw to have to introduce such a vagary into the story, but the M.V. *Victoria*, seventy feet of ice-breaking, oceangoing tugboat embarrassingly named for me, is Parker's alter ego. It is his mistress and his psychiatrist as well, and there is no question in my mind that it is a lot cheaper and less disruptive to family life than either of those would be.

In 1973 he decided that he needed a tugboat. "I have a large family; I need a large boat," he said, and bought one. The fact that it was nearly derelict disturbed him not a bit, and by June of 1976, with himself and every other available family member but me working on it every available moment of every available day, it was almost in seagoing condition again. Even I had stopped calling it an albatross.

On the tug that noon, painting away together through Parker's lunch hour, he and Sam had companionably solved the problem of a summer job, and, as Parker said to me, "If it seems too much for him working on the wharf, I can always find something for him to do on the tug."

"Or he could even work for Rozzie and me unpacking the china from Mother and Daddy's house in town once we start moving," I said.

"Sure, but he wouldn't like it as well," Parker said, and I gave him a friendly kick.

So another summer got under way, and Parker and I, determined that it should be just as normal as it could possibly be for everyone, tried not to dwell on the subject of Sam's sickness. Outside of Bill and Rozzie and Dottie, only Unkie (and we presumed Dana, his wife) knew that a heart transplant was ultimately Sam's only hope, and we didn't talk about it among ourselves. Parker started crooning his annual summer dirge, "Oh, it's a long long haul from June to September," and Rozzie and I worked at packing up the house in town. Begrudging every minute we had to spend away from the Cape, we would return there at night to hear an awesome list of festivities that the children were organizing. Pokie busied himself lining up bands, while Tina fell in love, Louise was fallen in love with, and Alix announced that things were so boring at home that she thought she'd go to a horse camp for two weeks.

The C & P Painting Company reported dutifully to the wharves to work, but after the afternoon that the uniforms were bought, Sam retreated back into quietness. In his boxcar-unloading days, he would come home at night either black or white, depending on whether charcoal or calcium chloride had been the product of the day, to stand in the middle of the kitchen in everyone's way, flexing his muscles and assuring Alix that he could crush her to pieces with one bare hand. After that he had always said, "C'mon, Al, race ya to the pool," and the two of them were out the door.

Now he would drag into the house with barely a grunted hi and collapse in a chair in the living room or on his bed in the back room. But unfailingly, at six thirty, he would get up and progress slowly to the telephone in the dining room to plan his evening. Getting supper in the kitchen, I rapidly learned to dread that moment when, in a forced, overly cheerful voice, he would say into the phone, "Hi, Fred," — or Craig, or Mike, or whomever he had dialed — "what's up? Yeah, the Whalers' Club at eight. See ya." Even Pokie, who was the acknowledged social lion of the family, and Tina, who ran a close second, had their nights off, and three or four nocturnal forays a week had always sufficed for Sam before.

"Sam," I would say, coming in from the kitchen, "don't you think it would be a good idea to stay home and rest up just for once? You don't have to hit the bars every night, you know," and in return I would be fixed with a scathing glance and a "Christ, Mum, I'm seventeen."

The Fourth of July fell on Sunday in 1976. Pokie was to produce a keg of beer and Uncle Bill the toasting book that Tina had made him for Christmas. With the number of great American Patriots to be drunk to, the party had to be scheduled to begin by eight o'clock in the morning, and costumes, Bill decreed, were in order. Every half hour during the entire day there were to be parades around the pool led by himself with his bass drum.

Although Ruthie and Malcolm were missing because the Coast Guard needed his services to usher the Tall Ships into New York Harbor, and Charlie and the Trinity crew had rowed their way that day into the finals of the Henley, the rest of the troops and myriad friends began to assemble on schedule.

Alix, carried away by a pronouncement from Uncle Bill that she should always be second in line in the parades because she played "a mean flute," used an entire bottle of ketchup on a handkerchief to make herself a part of "The Spirit of '76." Pokie and Sam attired themselves in neckties bearing the same motif, but as they wore nothing else other than painting hats and bathing trunks, they presented a bizarre salute to the nation. Along with his immaculate khakis, white shirt, and bass drum, Uncle Bill wore a six-inch-wide, five-foot-long, white necktie bedecked with red and blue stars and stripes, while Parker, uncostumed, shook his head from the minute he got up in the morning.

"Someone will have to stay sober around here," he announced, "and it doesn't look to me as if anyone else is planning to."

Messages drifting down to the cottage from the pool

seemed to indicate that there was some trouble opening the keg. The day was muggy and the paper stars Tina was gluing on her Statue of Liberty costume kept falling off, so in actuality it was closer to nine, while I was washing the breakfast dishes in the kitchen, that I heard the rolling of the bass drum, the tootling of Alix's flute, and Uncle Bill bellowing from the pool, "The Bi-cen-tennial is officially here. We shall drink our first toast to General George Washington!"

My white running shorts, an old red rowing shirt of Malcolm's, and a blue apron seemed hardly patriotic enough for such an occasion, so I ran out to Sam and Charlie's room and hastily surveyed the ceiling and the walls, from which hung the trophies of childhood. Dismissing the elk antlers from Wyoming as too heavy and Charlie's sixth-grade strong-man suit as inappropriate, I ended up torn between Sam's fourth-grade Viking hat, complete with horns, and an Indian headdress of unknown origins. I decided on the headdress and, shaking the remnants of winter mouse droppings from the feathers, I put it on my head and started back through the house to go up to the pool.

In the dining room I bumped into Sam, who was struggling out the door with the huge old maple music box that has lived at the cottage for ages. I move it once a year when I clean in the spring, and it must weigh ninety pounds.

"Put it down, Sam," I cried. "It's too heavy!"

"Pokie told me to bring it up to the pool," he said, continuing out the door. "They wanna play 'The Stars and Stripes Forever.'"

"Put it down, Sam," I repeated. "If Pokie wants it, he can come down and get it himself."

I don't remember any of the children ignoring a deliberate order of mine before or since, but Sam gave me an angry glare and kept right on going, bent almost double under the weight of the music box. I tore past him up to the pool, me and my feathers interrupting the drum, the flute, and Pokie, presiding over the beer keg.

"Damn it, Pokie," I exploded, "you go down and get that music box. It's too heavy for Sam."

"Oh, God, Mother," Pokie said in bored tones, "stop babying him," but he did leave the keg to help.

By nightfall the whole event had faded in the haze of a glorious Fourth. Charlie called from England to say that Trinity had won, and I had blocked out of my mind the picture of Sam laboring under the weight of the music box. In its place I put one of Tina, the Statue of Liberty, standing silver-crowned, her torch held high, on the bow of the outboard while Pokie motored her two coves away to call on the neighbors.

I also tried, but less successfully, to forget what Dana had said to me before lunch. Thinking, incorrectly as it turned out, that Unkie had told her about Sam, I had asked her not to tell anyone outside the family how bad things were.

"Oh, no," she had gasped with genuine shock, drawing away from me. "Oh, no, I didn't know. Don't tell me any more."

I had been hurt and angry and had found myself, against all Mother's and Rozzie's rules, crying again.

It was a good thing that Monday was a holiday too, but by Tuesday we were all back in action organizing the 1940s costume party and dance that Louise and Pokie were giving on Saturday night. It was to be held at the Tea House, a little gray-shingled building that used to grace the tennis court between the cottage and my parents' summer house. Within my memory, tea had never been served in it, and in

1938 my maiden aunt had it removed to the land near the pond, where a brook runs through the property, and had it surrounded by a twelve-foot-high stone wall because she was, she said, "tired of views."

Inside the wall all is paved terrace and garden, peach trees, roses, and wisteria. A little bridge spans the brook and leads across to the Tea House itself. It is a truly secret garden, and Pokie and Louise, both singly and jointly, had been trying to give a party there for years. But Nanny, my maiden aunt, did not approve of anyone who took more than one drink, and it was no surprise to any of us after she died that every time the children planned a party at her Tea House, it rained. The weather report could be glowing, the heavens cloudless, but the minute the beer keg passed through the little green door in the stone wall, the heavens opened.

Daddy, however, regularly took more than one drink, and after he died Pokie and Louise were inspired to try again.

"Maybe Grampa will tell Nanny to knock it off, Pokie," Louise said hopefully.

"Of course he will," Pokie assured her. "I can just hear him — 'Goddammit, Esther, let the damned kids have their goddamned party.' "

He must have done just that, because beer, gin, whiskey, and rum all passed through the little green door without so much as a cloud scudding across the full moon that shone the night of the tenth.

The dance began at nine, and the band (with the unlikely name of Shorty Hill and the Longhaulers) was indeed, as Pokie had assured us, a true 1940s type, complete with "thrush." "Sentimental Journey" was wafting sweetly over the walls as we adults and an assortment of our favorite forties-type friends arrived at the Tea House about ten.

Rozzie, who never throws anything away, was not only garbed in her complete going-away-from-her-wedding costume but had unearthed enough of her old evening dresses to attire at least ten of the female guests. From the garish smiles bestowed upon us by a majority of the ladies at the party, it was evident that her 1940s lipsticks had been put to good use as well. The Japanese lanterns glowed, the candles on the round tables we had set up burned brightly beneath the wisteria, and Rozzie said to me, "The children must remember to thank Grampa."

We had all agreed that dancing rather than drinking was to be encouraged during the evening, because the brook, edged by tiered stone walls, ran directly through the middle of the dance floor, but no one was surprised when a young gentleman, white tie and tails dripping, emerged from the brook, the victim of a misstepped fox-trot. It was dark enough and crowded enough to make positive identification of anyone at a given moment a little tricky, but it was just about then that I first spotted Sam.

His grandfather's evening clothes had passed to him by law of size and shape, although a good many safety pins compensated for the difference in their waistlines, and he and Fred and a gloriously unfaded 1940s girl were posing for Uncle Bill's camera. They seemed blissfully unaware that they were teetering on the very edge of the bridge over the brook. Freddie was holding up a bottle of Tanqueray gin in his right hand while his left was draped over the girl's shoulder. On her other side stood Sam, with his right arm around her, a bright yellow daisy in his teeth, and a Cupid's bow of violent red lipstick on his cheek. He looked deliriously happy, but he was drenched with perspiration, and the left side of his dinner jacket near his heart was visibly and wildly going in and out.

"Parker," I said, looking up at him nervously, "why is Sam's coat doing that and why is he sweating so? I've never seen him do that before."

We were standing in the doorway of the stone wall, and Uncle Bill turned his camera away from Sam to photograph us. In the picture, wearing the dress Mother wore at my wedding, I look timid and frightened, and I was.

I got up at six thirty the next morning. Including the little building next to the cottage where Pokie sleeps, the Poole summer household has beds, using the word loosely, for fourteen, and I sensed, as I left our own, that the remainder were full. As I crept quietly from doorway to doorway, sight confirmed sense; even the old wicker couch on the front porch was occupied.

In the bottom bunk of Sam's bed, Moriah, the dog, was draped disconsolately over an inert body with whom she had been forced to share the mattress she normally claimed as her own, while above her Sam lay on his back. He wasn't snoring, but the strangest sounds of breathing I had ever heard were coming from his throat. I'd gotten so used to his perpetual cough, terrible as it was, that I barely thought about it anymore. To me it was just an accepted — though still medically unexplained — part of his disease. But his breathing that morning terrified me. He would gasp in for breath and then exhale much later with a dreadful rattling noise. From time to time he seemed to stop breathing altogether, and then the blankets covering him would begin to heave and pulse over his chest just the way his dinner jacket had the night before.

I went back to the kitchen trembling. "Oh, my God," I kept muttering to myself, "what is happening? Why does he do that?"

I took a cup of coffee up to Parker, and he was comforting. "You'd breathe pretty queerly too if you'd drunk what he drank last night," he said. "He and Fred polished off that whole fifth of gin, and he didn't come in until six this morning. He woke me up crashing around downstairs."

I never saw Sam happy again all summer after that night. He went to work every day, and God knows he kept on going out every night, but he'd given up tennis, which he loved, because, he said, "it's such a hassle to get all changed to play," and he'd given up swimming even on weekends, because "the water's too cold." On Sunday noon he would drag up to the pool for the picnic, always with a friend in tow, and, bypassing lunch, he would sit, silent and remote with a towel over his eyes, in a chair removed from the thick of things. Whatever the temperature — and it was hot that summer — he invariably wore a Shetland sweater and over that, quite often, a heavy flannel shirt. The friend would swim with the other kids and eat along with the rest of us, but I noticed that whoever it was always sat in a chair near Sam and looked at him questioningly from time to time as if to say, "Is everything all right? Do you want me to shove off now so you can get some rest?"

To my own amazement, I even began to contemplate breaking the cardinal rule of motherhood and asking Freddie, or Craig of the C & P Painting Company, if they were worried about Sam, but I abandoned the idea almost immediately. The laws of teenage friendship could have allowed me at most only a "Gee, Mrs. Poole, I don't know."

When a friend from Kent arrived on a bus from Boston on the hottest day of the summer only to be picked up by Sam and driven back to Boston to go to a Red Sox game, I began, as the children say, to blow my cool.

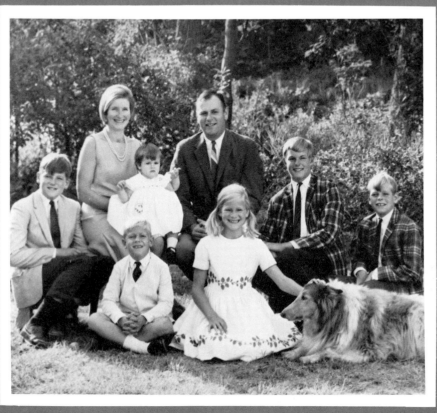

The Poole family in 1965, the Week
before disaster struck and
Pokie fell in the cesspool

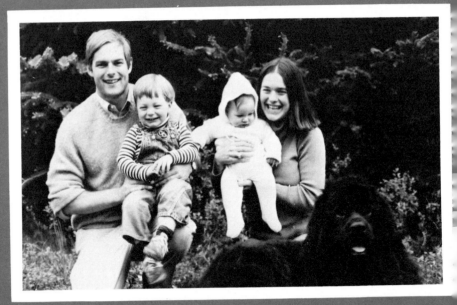

Malcolm and Ruthie with their
children and dog

Pokie in Adriatic waters,
doing his thing

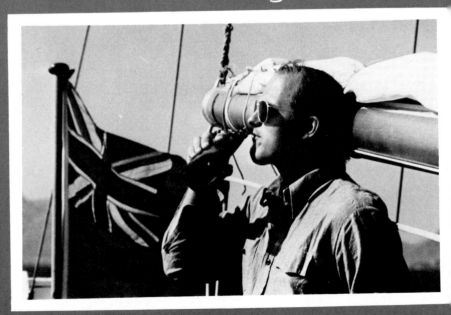

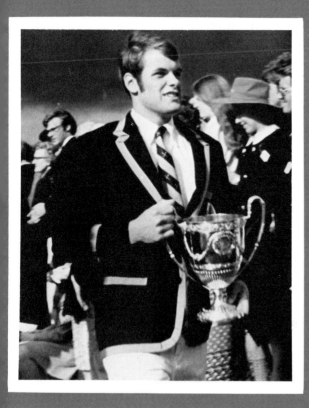

Charlie at
Henley, 1972,
holding the
bottom half
of the cup
won by the
Kent crew

Niece Louise
and dog
Oliver

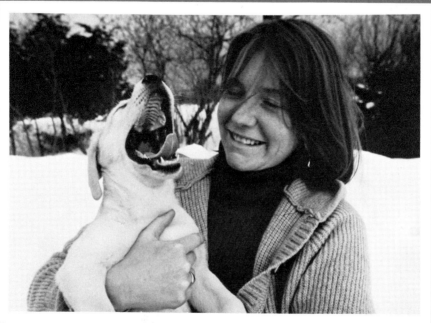

Tina

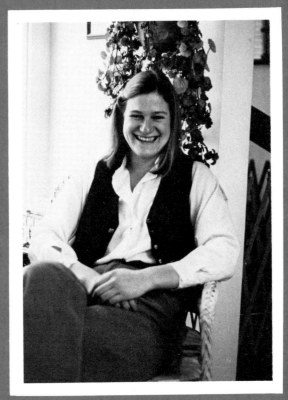

Alix with
nephew Gussie
(left) and niece
Beth

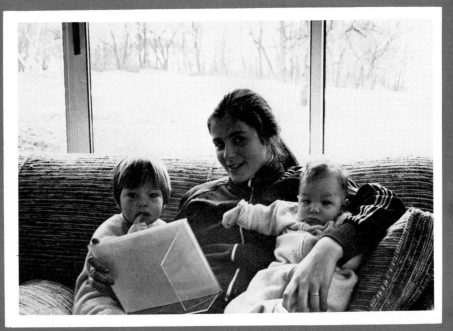

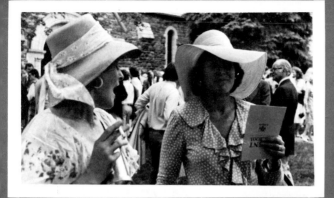

The Snoop
Sisters, Aunts
Vic (left) and
Roz

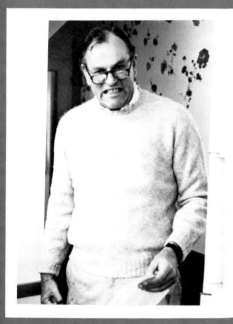

Parker snarling

Uncle Bill at
the start of
the family
Bicentennial
Celebration

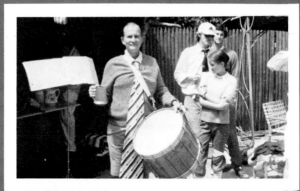

Dottie

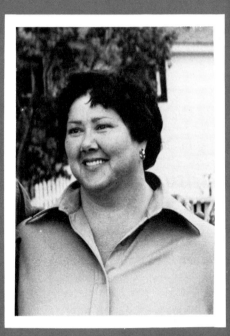

Dana (left) and Unkie

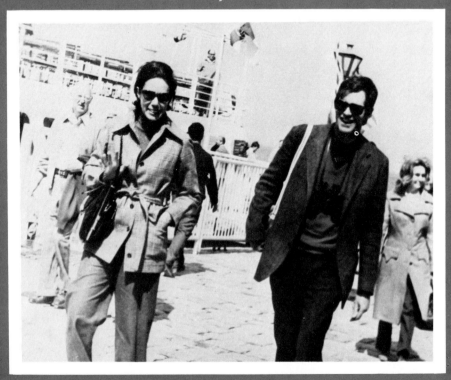

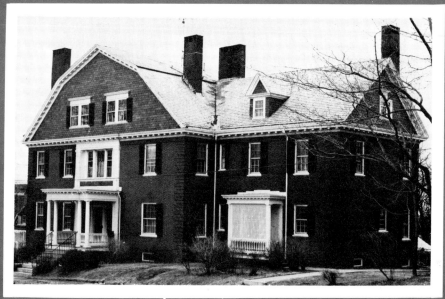

My Parents' house in Portland, where We
spent the Winter Sam got Sick

Moriah leading a friend to Camp Bruin

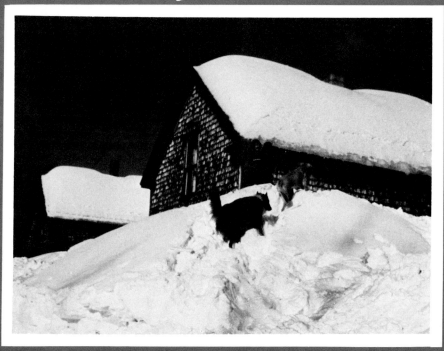

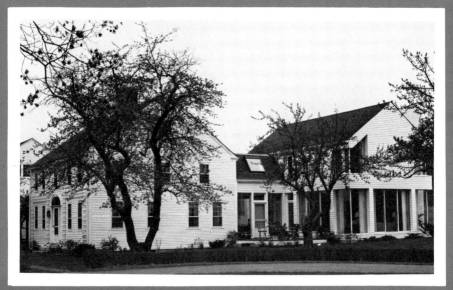

The Cape Elizabeth house, new addition at right

A view of our summer cottage from our winter house, 500 feet away

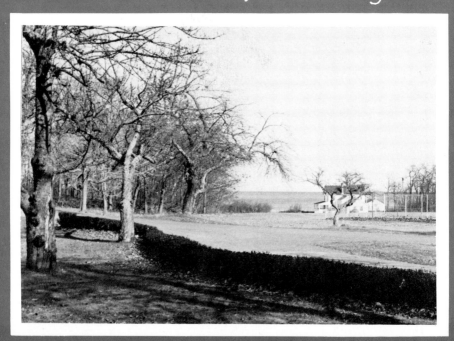

"Why?" I demanded when Sam got home the next day.

"He talks a lot," Sam said, "and it makes me so tired to listen. It's just easier to do something."

Two days later, looking like death warmed over, he insisted on going to Camden, two hours down the coast, to visit the girl who'd captivated him the night of the Tea House party. When he got home twenty-four hours later looking worse, I had inwardly reached the end of my tether.

I reached it outwardly the next night at dinner when Pokie asked Sam if he wanted to go to town for a beer. Against my protests that he looked like hell and, what's more, hadn't even touched his dinner, Sam said, "Sure."

I was cross, and I got up from the table and started to clear it, launching simultaneously and with vociferous enthusiasm into my traditional evening lament that begins, "I have so much to do and so little help from anyone."

It was poor Tina who inadvertently stuck her head in the lion's mouth. The children regularly tease me about the lament, and normally I let them, but that night, as Tina rose from the table to help me as she regularly does, she was foolhardy enough to say, "Poor Mum! What about all those cleaning ladies?"

I looked at her for one split second, and then all hell broke loose. Unlike Sam, I did not inherit my father's saintly face, but I do possess, to my shame, his most unholy temper. Over the years, however, I have more or less abandoned rages as a way of life, having concluded that they are exhausting, time-consuming, and quite futile as a means of attracting Parker's attention. I did not reflect on those conclusions that night. I shrieked, I screamed, I scooped up all the dirty laundry piled up next to the washing machine in the kitchen and hurled it at the children. I disowned everyone present, beginning with Tina, who'd made the remark, and following in rapid order with Pokie, who'd suggested the beer in town, Sam, who'd said he'd join him, and ending with a recently returned Charlie, on general principles. Alix was lucky enough to have departed for her horse camp. I stamped out of the kitchen with the dog in my wake, pausing only in the living room to announce to Parker, who was calmly reading the newspaper, that I was "finished, through, and leaving for good," and crashed out through the porch door. It was dark and it was raining, and I stumbled up the field toward the tennis court with Moriah, sobbing out to her the entire catalogue of my woes. It began and ended with Sam, and an hour later when I got back to the house I was dripping wet but, thanks to Moriah, unburdened and back in my senses.

The next day Dottie, who was on vacation, called me up. "What's going on over there?" she demanded. "Christina came to my apartment this morning, and she thinks you've flipped your lid. You've got to tell the other kids about Sam so they can help and not be pulling the other way."

Dottie only tells us things she thinks we have to know, and Parker agreed with her when he came home that night. Sam was at Freddie's for dinner, and we told Pokie and Charlie and Tina that Sam would never be well again. When we got to the heart transplant and Parker said, "It's the only hope he has left," it was an agony to watch their faces.

Pokie went absolutely ashen. "I didn't know," he said. "I had no idea. I'd never have asked him to carry that music box," and Charlie said, "I hadn't seen him since May. When he breathes at night, it's like listening to a volcano, but I didn't say anything."

Tina flung her arms around me, and the next morning, after she had left for work, I found a note on my bureau. Parenthetically, Tina is inaccurately referred to as "the elderly ugly daughter," and the note said:

Dear Mama,
 Take care of yourself, I love you more than I can say.

Love you,
E. U. D

Malcolm and Ruthie came the next weekend, and we told them. Dottie had, as usual, been right. Sam now had five fervent new watchdogs, but they barked and growled around him unheeded. In vain, Pokie and Charlie and Tina yawned and guessed they'd "stay in tonight." The three of them never got more rest, but every night at six thirty Sam would drag over to the telephone, and I would hear the two words I'd grown to hate: "What's up?"

As time progressed, Mother's warning via Rozzie that "crying won't help" fell on deaf ears. Sam flatly refused to be helped at all, and, although I didn't dare tell Rozzie, after the chores of the day were done about four and before the evening ones began about five, I started disappearing for a walk with Moriah, my dog psychiatrist. She offered the fields as her couch, and I would sit down on a hummock with my arms around her while she patiently listened to what had gone wrong with Sam since the day before, and never submitted a bill. I would return home more or less sane and with enough jaw-clenched courage to face the next "What's up?"

It was at the end of July that Sam began to complain of what he called "the full feeling." "I can't eat any more supper," he would say. "I feel full," and, knowing that he couldn't be from the amount of food he'd eaten, we were bewildered. He started vomiting too.

Parker and I drove over to New Hampshire on Saturday morning at the end of July to bring Alix home from her camp. It was a dreary day, and Sam was still asleep when we left. We got home that afternoon just in time to turn on the TV to watch Charlie and the Trinity crew on ABC's "Wide World of Sports," but no sooner had the sequence finished than Rozzie called up.

"Sam's on his way down to the cottage," she said, "but something's wrong with him. He came up here to watch Charlie with us, but the whole rest of the day he just sat in the rocking chair in front of the gas heater at the cottage, shivering as if it were January."

He was just coming in the door as I hung up, and, sick or not, seeing his older brother on national television had elated him.

"I'm Charlie Poole," he said in a great deep voice, squaring his shoulders and striding toward us in imitation of his brother's moment of video glory. "I'm from Portland, Maine. I stroke the boat."

Sam looked so thin and so gray that it was hard to imagine that he had ever been strong enough to pick up an oar, let alone row with one, and no sooner had we laughed and said, "Oh, Sam, you're so mean," than he forgot his joy in Charlie and fled to the back room. We could hear him throwing up and rushed out to see what was wrong.

"Something I ate," he said when he was finished, tossing it off.

The next Friday night something happened that couldn't be tossed off. Parker and I were talking in the kitchen before dinner. Sam was outside the kitchen door, tinkering with an old outboard motor that Pokie had given him, and suddenly we saw him coming back toward the house looking frightened and sick.

"What is it?" Parker asked.

"I lifted up the motor," he said, "and I felt so sick. It must have been the fumes."

He sat down on a chair for a second, and then suddenly he said, "My left hand's getting all tingly. It feels numb."

I rushed over to him and put my hand on his back, and he said, "It's going up my arm. I can feel it," and his words began to sound thick, and he spoke without moving his lips and as if he weren't moving his tongue.

"It's all swollen. My tongue's all swollen," he moaned and heaved himself up out of the chair and staggered toward his room. He couldn't get to the bathroom. At the doorway he started to vomit, and it was all clear liquid. There was no solid matter in it at all.

He was still vomiting when Parker finally got him leaning over the toilet. I stood beside Sam, pressing a wet washcloth on his forehead with one hand and trying to rub his back with the other. His shoulder blades stuck out through his T-shirt like bare bones. The retching finally turned into dry heaves, and his whole body was shaking as he tried to support himself over the toilet.

"Parker," I said, "you've got to call Dr. Hall. This is the numbness he was talking about. You've got to call him right now."

He helped me lead Sam over to his bed, and together we helped him up to the top bunk. He lay there for a second, exhausted, and then he said, "Oh, my head hurts so and my eyes. All I can see is down this tunnel. Oh, it hurts so." Parker left the room to call the doctor.

Dr. Hall had left the hospital, but his receptionist, who

was familiar with Sam's problem, said she would get in touch with him at home and have him call us.

He did almost immediately. He was just on his way out for dinner and in a rush, he explained, "but just off the top of my head, I'd say it was a migraine headache. I wouldn't worry about it too much if I were you. We'll check him out next week, but another time don't try to call me at home. I'm not supposed to have private patients because of my connection with the hospital, you know. Just have him keep quiet and give him some aspirin."

Sam threw up the aspirin, and after that he lay motionless on his bed except when he became racked with another attack of dry heaves or his cough.

Back in the kitchen once Sam seemed to be resting more easily, I could see that Parker was angry. "Who are we supposed to call when something like this happens? When Sam had the catheterization in June, I thought Dr. Hall told us to call him if anything different happened. I'd like to know who the hell we're supposed to call!" he demanded of me, but I had no answer.

Sam went in on Monday to see Dr. Hall, and it seemed that the telephone diagnosis was entirely correct. His heart condition, we were assured, remained stable, and we were instructed to carry on as usual.

And we did carry on, but it wasn't easy because things never got any better. Sam seemed to grow thinner and colder and more miserable every day. The mucus he coughed up grew thicker, and often, when I cleaned his bathroom in the morning, I would notice that it was tinged with dark stains. The second migraine came the day after he saw Dr. Hall and was followed with precision by the third and the fourth and the fifth.

Dr. Hall had told us to call Tom Mansfield, our family

doctor, if the migraines recurred, and Tom made an appointment for Sam with a neurologist. The neurologist had him have an electroencephalogram to rule out the possibility of a brain disorder or a tumor, and it did, but once again poor Sam was confronted with a malady for which there appeared to be no cure. Migraines, we were told, are usually the direct result of tension. Sam was justifiably tense because of his heart condition, and, as long as he was, the migraines would probably continue.

"It must all be bottled up inside him then," I moaned to Parker, "because if anyone asked me to describe him, I'd say 'limp' was more like it than 'tense.'" Dr. Mansfield prescribed a capsule which Sam was to put under his tongue the instant he felt the onset of a migraine, and he did as instructed, but to no avail. The numbness, the vomiting, the tunnel vision, and the pain of migraine were upon him before the capsule could start to work.

Every morning I would nervously ask him, when he appeared in the kitchen determined to go to work, "Do you feel all right, Sam? Is it any better today?" and I usually got a slight nod or an "I'm okay." One morning about a week after his first migraine, though, I met him coming out of the bathroom off his bedroom. I asked him the by-then-traditional question, and instead of the nod he said, "Oh, Mum, it just hurts so to get out of bed. I wish I could get up in the morning and just say, 'I feel good.' You know, like it's going to be a nice day."

I could only swallow hard and pat his poor thin shoulder and say, "Oh, darling, I do too."

We rarely sit down for dinner in August without one or two visiting firemen, and that August was no exception. Sam usually sat down for dinner with us, but before the meal was half over, and without touching his plate, he invariably fled to the bathroom to throw up. Parker and I would both leap up from the table, but he, who had always left vomiting children to me before, would more often than not say now, "You stay here, I'll go with him," and I would stay behind, trying to carry on the dinner conversation as if nothing were amiss.

Through the thin beaverboard walls of the cottage would come the sounds of poor Sam's hideous, gasping retches, and I would say brightly to the visitor, "Oh, I can't tell you how grand it is to have you here."

It was a great relief to have a doctor on the premises — my cousin Parker Vanamee, a physiologist at Memorial Hospital in New York, finally arrived at the Cape for his annual vacation. Poor P.V. (as we all call him to distinguish him from my Parker, P.P.) endured a busman's holiday from start to finish that summer. The very night he arrived, we appeared at his house to bring him up to date on Sam. When we got to the heart transplant, he gave a low whistle and shook his head.

"Oh, boy," he said. "I wouldn't go that route unless I absolutely had to."

Two nights later Parker was out of town on business, and I went up to Bill and Rozzie's to have a drink with Bill's sister and her husband, another doctor. Bill and Rozzie had told him about Sam, and his advice to me was gentle and kind, but very firm. If he were in our position, under no circumstances would he ever consider a heart transplant for Sam. He knew a man who had had severe cardiomyopathy since childhood and was now well over forty. "Of course," he said, "he's never done anything physical at all. He collected something, I think — stamps, perhaps — but nothing physical."

I thanked him politely and flew home in tears. How could I make Sam live to be forty and collect stamps when I couldn't even get him to stay home one night a week unless he was vomiting or having a migraine? Only the night before I'd gone out to his room to see if he was all right after he'd stopped throwing up, and he'd said, with tears running down his cheeks and his fists clenched on either side of him as he lay on the bed, "Mum, oh, Mum, I don't want to be sick," and he'd gotten up the next morning to go to work.

He had started coming home earlier from partying, though. He'd been gone only an hour one night when he reappeared looking shaken and exhausted.

"I got sick," he said. "I just ordered one lousy drink, and I got sick before I even drank it. I blew everything in the men's room for twenty minutes, and I went back and drank it then, but I hadn't even touched it before."

And when I asked him why he'd drunk it at all, he protested impatiently, "Christ, Mum, I had to pay for it."

He and Craig had finished the wharves and the tugboat by then and were working for Rozzie and me, unpacking china from the house in town. It was only later I found out that Sam kept an empty packing box beside him at all times to throw up into and that every night he and Craig would drive it and its contents to the town dump to dispose of it. It was not until later too that I found out he could no longer walk from one bar to another even if the two were only separated by a block. His right side hurt him so whenever he took a step that he had to clutch it in order to walk at all.

But I didn't know those things then, and, with all the china unpacked, Sam demanded to know what job he and Craig could do next. It was late on a Monday afternoon toward the end of August, and Rozzie and I were preparing to depart for New York the next morning at dawn. We abandoned our packing to try feverishly to think of a project that would keep him occupied but not exhausted until we came home and finally settled on painting the trim of the Tea House. We selected from a paint chart at the hardware store a color which appeared to be a cheerful yellow and departed for our trip, instructing Sam to "do what you feel like. Don't push yourself. It's no crisis job." Not until our plane landed in New York did Rozzie discover that she had one brown and one black shoe on and no wallet. Although both of us are given to blaming anyone but ourselves for such annoyances, it is a measure of Sam's aunt's affection for him that she never once attributed her dishevelment to his interruptions.

We came home two days later. Sam was in bed with a terrible migraine, and the trim of the Tea House was half painted a color which was then — and still is — best described as "vomit yellow."

When she came to work the next day, Dottie filled me in on what had happened, since Sam had been too miserable to talk the night before. He and Craig, she said, had painted on Tuesday and on Wednesday, but when she got to the cottage on Thursday morning about nine thirty, he was in the bathroom throwing up. He couldn't stop, he kept missing the toilet, and, as she put it, "the whole damn john was knee-deep in orangeade." He told her he'd gone to the Tea House about eight with a full pitcher of it to share with Craig, but by eight thirty he'd been so thirsty he'd drunk the whole thing alone. "He said it just started coming up then," she explained, "and no sooner did he stop throwing up than the headache came and lasted the whole day."

"He's still got it," I said. "He's out there in his room in

bed now. All he's told me is how tired he got and how tiresome it was to mix the paint, but I don't care what he says after this, Dottie, he can't work anymore."

Sam never talked about working again. Even after the headache let up, he was so sick he could barely get up. P.V. came down to the cottage to check him over, but, like the other doctors, he assured us that he couldn't detect anything alarming going on in Sam's chest.

"Talk about adding insult to injury," he said to me. "Here's the poor kid with a bad heart, and the Lord has to send him migraines just to be sure he's really miserable. 'Tain't fair, Beek-Beek," he finished, calling me by the name he had bestowed upon me when I was sixteen.

It seemed impossible to me that day that I had ever been sixteen, but he was right; t'weren't fair. Sam alternated between his bed and the living-room couch all that weekend, and on Monday morning when I woke up at four o'clock I found Parker already sitting on the edge of the bed, looking out the window at the ocean. The tide was almost low.

"I feel as if everything that's normal in our lives and everything I've ever believed in is ebbing away with that tide," he said. "I look at Sam and I know he's sick, and, even though the doctors all say it has nothing to do with his heart, I don't believe it. I don't believe it for a minute, and I'm not going to sit back and let him go out with that tide."

Chapter Five

Parker's determination was contagious, but by breakfast time I had sunk back into my slough of despond.

"How are you going to keep Sam from going out with the tide when we don't even know what doctor to take him to for what anymore?" I complained over my fifth cup of coffee. "We've gone from Mansfield, to Dr. Hall, to Wakely, back to Dr. Hall, and now, for God's sake, we're back at square one with Dr. Mansfield again. Sam's head is sick and his stomach is sick and his heart is sick, and where the hell are you going to start? And," I finished, almost in tears, "whoever you do take him to will only say there isn't anything that can be done anyway."

"I thought it all out when I was in the shower," Parker said. "I've decided the hell with Dr. Hall. I went to high school with Tom Mansfield, and I'm just going to tell him he's got to do something about Sam."

Tom did. After Parker and I, with P.V. along for professional support, described the extent of Sam's miseries to him in his office that afternoon, he said, "Well, I guess we'd better put him in the hospital and run some tests on him."

"Thank God," I said to P.V., as we drove home together to the Cape, and then I said to myself, "Oh, my God!" It was going to be January all over again. The two interior decorators were returning the next afternoon for a three-day visit to check on the progress of the new house, and they were bringing their children with them. On Friday, after they left, five Perrys were coming from Kent for the weekend.

"I'm going to kill myself," I said to Rozzie when I got home. "There's no other way out. The ladies have already left for Maine for their vacation so I can't tell them to come later, and here's Sam going into the hospital tomorrow. I'm going to kill myself right now."

Rozzie understands hyperbole. To everyone's despair, it's how we cope with all minor crises. *"Calma, calma,"* she said benignly in the vestigial accents of a long-past trip to Italy. "It will all work out," and it did, but mostly thanks to her.

There are moments in my life when, with a smile, I could annihilate Rozzie, such as when it's my turn to wash first in the sink at Camp Bruin and she's snuck ahead of me. At times like that I have sadistically hoped that her Erno Laszlo face creams may have frozen overnight. However, she earned herself many future firsts at Bruin's sink with unfrozen Erno that week.

She entertained the decorators — and their children — while I visited Sam, and she visited Sam while I trailed along behind them through the new house. I watched them mix paints with the painter, plan valances with the drapery woman, and explain to the paperhanger that "those daffodils should look as if they're just peeping over the top of that beam. Yes, just like that!" I admired everything, but all that registered in my mind was: When can I decently leave and get back to Sam?

He had a terrible migraine with a violent attack of vomiting his first night in the hospital, and, when I went in on Wednesday morning, he was having an intravenous feeding to combat dehydration. By Thursday the IVs were done, but he had acute diarrhea. The full feeling in his stomach, however, was mercifully disappearing.

"Geez, it oughta be," he grumbled to me. "I had the runs all night, and I've been to the can about twenty times this morning. It's funny, though, Mum. It's all this clear liquid just like when I throw up. It's just like water."

I could only shake my head, and we both lapsed into the silence that was getting to be our new means of communication.

The interior decorators and their children tactfully departed early Friday morning, and Dottie told me she'd get things ready for the Perrys. "You're only in the way when I'm cooking anyway," she said.

I sat with Sam most of the day. I sat with him through the quiz programs until his lunch came, which he didn't touch, and through the soap operas until his supper came, which he didn't touch either. At one point in the morning, I had gone downstairs to the hospital canteen to get him a Coke and had run into a friend of mine. Over a cup of coffee, she had asked me, "What are they going to do about Sam's heart, then, Vicky?" and I had just looked at her stupidly and said, "Nothing. There's nothing they can do."

The dreadful matter-of-factness of the words stayed with me all day, and when I tried to banish them, they were replaced by lines from a Hilaire Belloc poem I'd once thought uproariously funny and had regularly recited to the children —

Physicians of the Utmost Fame
Were called at once; but when they came
They answered, as they took their Fees,
"There is no Cure for this Disease.
Henry will very soon be dead."

It was the most dismal of days until Ruthie and Malcolm appeared in the doorway. They were just starting a two-week vacation, and Ruthie proclaimed before she'd even gotten into the room, "We're having a baby!" Her blue eyes were dancing and her brown hair was flying, and for the first time since he had been in the hospital, Sam sat up without the slightest evidence of effort.

"Hey, great, Ruthie! I'll be Uncle Sam. Mum can buy me an Uncle Sam suit at Brooks."

Tom Mansfield gave Sam his walking papers that night too. He went over the results of the tests with us and with Parker, who'd come by then. There had been some evidence of slight liver dysfunction, and some small electrolytic imbalance was present in Sam's blood chemistry, but, he said, "Today's tests indicate that things are getting back to normal. It seems to be the rest he's had that did the trick. We haven't had to give him any diuretics at all or anything to stimulate his heart, so on the whole I can only presume he's been doing too much. We will start him now on low dosages of both as a preventive measure, and he can go home tomorrow, but I think he ought to quit working."

"Don't worry," I said. "He already has."

The Perrys with their three children came that night about nine. "Why didn't you tell us not to come?" they exclaimed when they heard that Sam was in the hospital.

We were sitting in the living room having a welcoming drink with them. The kids had gone up to the pool with

Alix for a welcoming swim, and Parker said, "No. We wanted you to come so we could talk to you face to face before Sam goes back to Kent. We don't know what we're getting you into."

"You see," I said, "Sam's not going to be well again and we don't know what's going to happen. He wants to go back more than anything in the world, and we want him to if he can, but do you want him?"

"Of course we do. We need him," Hart said, but his face was as stricken as the children's had been when we told them. After Parker explained that a heart transplant was probably somewhere down the road for Sam, Hart just took a deep breath and came over and gave me a hug. "Look, he's got Kent School to back him up," he said. "How can he lose?"

Parker and I brought Sam home from the hospital the next morning to have him greeted with true Kent spirit by a banner stretching across the whole front of the cottage saying, WELCOME HOME, SAM. An ersatz brass band, comprised of five Perrys and six Pooles armed with all my pots, pans, and kitchen utensils, was emitting dreadful noises in front of it, but no sooner had Sam kissed Fran Perry and grasped Hart's hand with a "God, it's great to see you, Mr. Perry," than he cursed. "Oh, Christ," he said, "I'm getting a migraine."

After the headache subsided that afternoon, however, he really did seem better, and a whole week passed with uncommon calm. He refused to eat on the grounds that the full feeling might come back if he did, but he assured me, when he went off to one end-of-summer party or another, that he'd abandoned drinking on the same grounds, and I tried to relax about him.

The Saturday before Labor Day he went to an afternoon

"beer baseball" game, then to Sugarloaf that night for a concert, before returning Sunday to go to another clambake with the Tea House girl and her family. He told me that he felt fine when he came home that night, but he fell asleep on the living-room floor, holding on to his right side as if he had a stomachache, and I had a dreadful time getting him up to go to bed.

Although Labor Day ranks a lowly fourth after Christmas, New Year's, and the Fourth of July as a favorite family holiday, its prestige in 1976 rose to a new high. Parker's tugboat was to make her maiden voyage. Family, friends, and friends of friends came to watch or to crowd on board for the great event, and, amid cheers and shouts, Parker slowly — and, I'm sure, nervously — propelled the M.V. *Victoria* out of her slip and into Portland Harbor. Sam was holding on to the bowline, and as he heaved it back up onto the wharf I said to Tina, "Isn't it marvelous. He really does look much better than he did before the hospital."

He even ate some lunch that noon, but when we got home that night, he collapsed again on the living-room floor and fell asleep watching TV. Parker, triumphant over his day, had gone up to bed, and no amount of my proddings and shakings could get Sam up.

"Oh, God, I'm too tired," he'd moan. "I just ache all over. Let me stay here, please, I feel so full."

I got him a pillow and some down puffs and let him, but it was my turn to have Parker find me sitting on the edge of the bed, looking out to sea, at four o'clock the next morning. As soon as he rolled over, I told him that Sam had the full feeling again.

"He can't go back to school like this," I said. "I'm not going to let him go anywhere until somebody looks at him."

I told Tom Mansfield the same thing on the phone later in the morning.

"You know," he said, "I've been thinking about this a lot, and I decided that if Sam's troubles came back after that stint in the hospital he should really have a cardiologist looking after him. Dr. Hall can't take him on as a regular patient because of his job with the hospital. So how would you feel if I asked Philip Wakely, who did his catheterization, to take over Sam's case?"

"Great," I said with more enthusiasm than I'd heard in my voice all summer. "That would be great." Only after I hung up did it occur to me to wish I'd asked why Dr. Wakely hadn't been officially appointed Sam's doctor after the catheterization in June.

We only had to wait until the next afternoon for Dr. Wakely to fit Sam in, and Sam went alone by choice to his office at three o'clock. For some reason that has never been clear in my mind, I was — of all unlikely places for me to be at three thirty in the afternoon — in the bathtub when the phone rang. Grabbing a towel, I slithered and slipped down the front stairs and reached over the banister and around the corner to pick up the telephone in the dining room. It was an awkward position in which to talk, but it was Sam.

"Dr. Wakely wants to speak to you," he said.

In the cottage, standing downstairs with nothing on but a towel is nerve-racking. You never know who might come in by any door, and I felt very foolish leaning over the banister, clutching my towel, and trying to comprehend what Dr. Wakely was saying. If I'd had more clothes on, I might better have defended my own opinions.

"I've checked Sam all over," he said, "and there's absolutely nothing to indicate that this problem of feeling full has anything to do with his heart. There is no congestion present at all. I'm afraid that, like the migraines, it's just a matter of nerves. I'm convinced that he's gotten acid indigestion from all the strain he's been under, and I've given him an antacid to take which will coat his stomach. It may well take care of the problem, but mostly he's got to try to stop worrying.

"Put yourself in his position, Mrs. Poole," he went on. "Think how you'd feel if you'd been told you had a heart condition like Sam's. I think that you and Mr. Poole have been remarkably calm about his problem on the whole, but you can't help but worry. And," he finished, "your worries about him must worry Sam. I'm going to ask you almost the impossible, to try not to be a nervous mother. He should go back to school and have a good year."

And all I said was, "Okay, Dr. Wakely." It bothered me, though, because if there was anything I was sure of, it was that I hadn't acted like a nervous mother with Sam. I couldn't sleep and food tasted pretty awful, but I know when I'm upsetting people and I knew I hadn't upset Sam. He'd have told me.

When I was getting supper that night, Sam was talking to Pokie in the dining room, and I heard him say, "Dr. Wakely says all I've got is acid indigestion, and he told Mum she's a nervous mother. He doesn't know her very well if he says that. God, she's never been nervous with any of us."

Listening to them discuss my foibles, like the time I made Charlie, with a broken but as yet un-X-rayed leg, go up three flights of stairs to get a pair of shoes to wear to the doctor's office, I wished I were a nervous mother. I wished I thought for one minute that all Sam had was acid indigestion caused by me, but I didn't. And Parker, when he came home that night, didn't either.

Sam was to leave for Kent on Saturday morning, and on Friday night I had a going-back-to-school dinner for him. He said he'd like Aunt Roz, Uncle Bill, and Louise to make it a party, with lobsters, clams, corn, and a going-away cake to eat, and I provided it all. We ate, in honor of the occasion, in the dining room, and only the absence of Charlie, who'd gone back to Trinity, and Ruthie and Malcolm, who'd gone back to New York, kept it from being a proper family party. Tina was taking her junior year in England, where courses, unlike Trinity's, started on the civilized date of October 1, and she was still at home.

The party started out festively until I inadvertently commented to Rozzie that the bill for my share of moving the furniture from our parents' house in town had come that day and was reasonable.

"Well, it shouldn't have been," Rozzie retorted. "I'm probably being billed for your share," and we were off.

Rozzie hadn't gotten her bill yet. If she had we would never have fought. With facts and figures before us, there would have been answers to any possible errors, and that would be a bore. It is only the challenge of the insoluble that piques Rozzie's mind toward argument. Normally our bickerings bore the children, are ignored by Bill, and only annoy Parker, but that night they infuriated him. We had mildly argued away through dinner and were halfway through the dishes, although nowhere nearly halfway through our fight, when Parker came bellowing out into the kitchen.

"Knock it off!" he roared, and, out of respect for his sensibilities, we repaired to the darkness of the yard outside the kitchen to continue. The children had departed for town, including Sam, who was having a last date with his Tea House love, and the sound of our voices drifting through the windows into the now-quiet living room incited Parker to a rage worthy of Daddy himself.

"Goddammit, shut up, you two," he exploded, crashing out of the kitchen door shaking his fist. "This was Sam's last night home. Here he may be dying, and all you two goddamned women can do is fight. You make me sick!" And he slammed back through the door.

"What does he mean Sam may be dying?" Rozzie demanded. "Dr. Wakely said he would go back to school and have a good year."

"Yes, but we don't believe it," I said, and she looked at me with total disbelief of her own and went home.

I was so mad at her that I couldn't clean up even inefficiently. I thought of the toast Sam had made to us during dinner and started to sniffle.

"Thank you all," he had said, standing up, his dinner untouched before him, raising a glass of milk to us. "Thank you all for putting up with the sick me this summer."

Parker had stomped his way up to bed, and at eleven when Tina came home from a date with Him (as we always refer to the girls' beaux), I was still wallowing around in a sea of lobster and clam shells, corncobs, and cake crumbs. She was a welcome change from Aunt Roz that night and a welcome change from acid indigestion, migraines, and cardiomyopathy as well. We sat at the kitchen table having a lovely time discussing Romance, but about twelve thirty we heard a car, and Sam came into the kitchen looking like death itself.

"Oh, God, I feel awful," he said. "Oh, I feel so awful. I didn't drink anything at all but, oh, God, I puked all over Exchange Street."

He was to leave for Kent the next morning at eight. At seven he staggered into our bedroom. "I've got a migraine," he said thickly between motionless lips.

"Go back to bed," Parker and I both said at once. "You can't go back to school," and he nodded his agreement.

About noon the migraine was gone, and he asked me to get him a glass of ginger ale. We had none, and, although I had vowed the night before never to go near Rozzie again and there had been no communication between the two houses all that morning, ginger ale for Sam precluded personal sentiment. I ran up the path to her house to find her sitting in a chair in the living room, staring out at the sea with tears running down her cheeks.

"Oh, Aunt Roz," I cried, running over to her and putting my arms around her, "what is it?"

"Uncle Bill has left me forever," she said.

"But he's always leaving you forever," I said. "When he left you forever in June, he was only gone for four hours."

"No, this time I know it's for good. He's even taken his bass drum. He was so mad at me last night after Uncle Parker blew up he came up here and just picked up his bass drum and left."

"I'll find him," I said, having no idea how I would. "Give me some ginger ale for Sam, and I'll find him."

Hearing that Sam was too sick to go back to school only added to her despair. As I left she walked out the sliding glass doors that face the sea as dramatically as though Uncle Bill were Rhett Butler and she was on her way back to Tara.

I ran back down the path to the cottage and bumped into

Sam, who was slowly progressing through the dining room to the living room. "Oh, Sam," I said, passing by him to go into the kitchen to open the ginger ale, "Uncle Bill has left Aunt Roz forever again, and no one knows where he's gone. How will I ever find him?"

"Why don't you look behind you?" he said. "Hello, Uncle Bill."

Uncle Bill was just coming in from the outside through the dining-room door with a large and very dark-looking drink in his hand. "I have left your sister forever," he announced to me.

"No, you haven't, Uncle Bill," Sam said. "I found you. You'll have to wait now till the next time," and he politely refused the rum Uncle Bill assured him was "just the thing for migraines, my boy."

That night Sam sat huddled up in a corner of the living-room sofa near the fireplace, bundled in a down puff, looking as defenseless as a little child. "He should go back to school and have a good year," I kept reminding myself all night, but it didn't do any good at all.

I was still in my nightgown and Parker was in his pajamas when we helped him pack his belongings into the old blue Volvo to drive to Hartford the next morning. Charlie was going to drive him over to Kent from there, but Sam looked so frail and sick and tired that it was all I could do to keep myself from saying, "Don't go. Oh, please, darling, don't go."

He waved a long thin arm out the window as he drove up the road from the cottage, and Parker put his arm around me. "The Volvo looks as sick as Sam does," he said. "I wonder if either one of them will get through this year."

The news from Kent that week was not reassuring. Hart

Perry called us Wednesday night. "Sam had a really bad time with one of those migraines today," he said. "It scared the heck out of us, and his roommate says he's been throwing up almost every night."

Sam had woken up with the migraine in the morning, according to Hart, but it had been such a struggle for him to get up that he'd missed early clinic. Father Rowins, one of the chaplains at the Boys' School, had found him absolutely glassy-eyed in a corridor, trying to find the master who authorized class absences.

"It really frightened Chuck," Hart said. "Sam looked so awful that he told him to forget about getting excused from classes and just go back to bed, but Sam kept on going till he found Don Gowan. He could hardly stand up by the time he did. We're going to keep a close eye on him, but how that poor kid can do his work is beyond me."

On Friday Parker and I drove to Kent to see Sam for ourselves and to leave off an old couch that he wanted for his room. We were going to spend the weekend with Bill and Georgie Bowers, our St. Kitts friends, who lived in Darien between hotel seasons. Although Kent was hardly on our way, neither of us could have gone near Connecticut without checking on Sam.

It was a quiet trip. Tina had had four impacted wisdom teeth extracted in the hospital on Wednesday, and her oral surgeon had told me when he discharged her on Thursday that the blood tests she had had before the surgery needed to be repeated by her own physician. "Things don't quite check out," he'd said.

"It's leukemia, I know it is," I had said to Rozzie after I'd tucked Tina into our bed and packed her unfamiliarly round face with bags of ice.

"It's not," Tom Mansfield speedily and emphatically assured me twenty-four hours later, but I was a basket case by the time we left for Kent. It was good to sit for five hours without talking.

At Kent we found Hart and sat with him in his office while someone went off to find Sam.

"Sam's doing a great job with Blue Key," he told us. "He's got a big outdoor dance with the Girls' School organized for this coming weekend, complete with a sound-and-light show, but I don't like the way he looks. I wish he'd complain or something, but he never does. George Griener, the school doctor, is keeping pretty close tabs on him, though, so try not to worry."

Seeing Sam made it hard not to. We went with him to his dormitory to unload the couch, and his roommate and some friends came piling out of the doorway to lift it out of the car before Sam could touch it. "Get outta the way, Poole," they said, and such uncommon courtesy at a boys' school didn't do a thing to ease my mind.

I went up the stairs to his room behind him. He started off quickly, as if there were nothing wrong, but half a flight up he was gasping for breath and hanging on to the railing for dear life.

"Call us," I said as we left, "if you think you'd rather come home. It's crazy to stay if you don't feel well."

"I feel fine," he said. "Remember what Dr. Wakely said, Mum. Don't be a nervous mother."

I laughed and kissed him good-bye, but Parker and I never said a word all the way to Darien, and I fought to keep back the tears. Bill and Georgie never had two drearier visitors, though they were too polite to complain.

We talked to Sam again on the telephone on Monday, September 27, and he complained that his cough was really getting bad and that he didn't "really feel all that well." He promised me that he'd go to Dr. Griener the next day, and he did, because at ten in the morning Hart called me.

"George Griener says he's detected some congestion in Sam's lungs, and he thinks he ought to go home and get it checked out," he said. "Can you come down?"

"Can I?" I said. "I'm on my way!"

I have never felt greater relief. Suddenly there was something wrong with Sam that nobody could call nerves. Finally somebody would have to do something.

I was taking Tina to Boston that day anyway because her plane flew from there to England, and by eleven I had called Parker, organized Alix with Dottie, thrown my night things in a bag, and departed for Kent via Boston. Hart had assured me that Fran would be delighted to have me spend the night with them.

"I'm not going to cry," I announced to Tina when I left her off with Him, who was going to take her out for dinner and put her on her plane, but I hugged her good-bye as if I'd never see her again.

"We'll write long letters, Mum, and it will be Christmas before we know it. I promise," she said, but I drove off with the held-back tears running down my cheeks. I've probably driven to Kent forty times since the day we first took Malcolm there, but that afternoon I made a misturn without realizing it, and it was getting dark by the time I finally got back on the right road. I turned on the headlights, but things kept getting darker and darker.

"Oh, God, I'm going blind," I wailed as I crept along at twenty miles an hour, and it wasn't until I was just outside of Kent that I realized that I still had my dark glasses on and had only turned on the parking lights. It was well after seven when, shaken and confused, I got to the Perrys. Sam was already there, but I didn't have a chance to talk to him alone till after dinner.

He was wretched about feeling so awful that I had had to come to Kent. "Oh, Mum," he said, "I just hate causing you all this trouble," and no amount of assurances that I wanted to be there and that it wasn't his fault seemed to help.

We were standing in Hart's study, and finally Sam looked at me and said point-blank, "Mum, what's wrong with me?"

"I don't know," I said, and the inadequacy of the words and the inhumanity of having to say them will stay with me forever.

The next morning was worse. Parker had called the night before and told me that he had talked to Dr. Wakely and that I was to deliver Sam to the hospital at two o'clock to be admitted for tests, so we left at eight o'clock for Portland. Sam insisted on driving more than half the way, and the car wove and lurched along the highway erratically. I bit my tongue and kept my eyes shut most of the time, and when I did open them to look at Sam, it was no comfort to find that his were almost closed. It was with great relief that I heard him say, "You wanna drive?"

That was all he'd said since we left Kent, and I don't think either of us said another word until we got almost to our exit on the Maine Turnpike. "Sam," I said then, "Daddy and I love you. Don't, please, shut us out of your life."

"I'm not, Mum," he answered, and his voice was choked. "I'm not. It's just I just said good-bye to my friends."

Doctor Griener's ear was faultless. There was indeed congestion in Sam's lungs, and in his intestines and liver as well. Before we got home to Portland, Dr. Wakely had arranged to have a specialist in gastrointestinal disorders check Sam over. He thought that perhaps the nervous indigestion had by this time produced an ulcer, but barium X-rays done the next morning ruled out any such possibility, and the gastrointestinal specialist gave a diagnosis of "visceral congestion."

Dr. Wakely immediately put Sam on stronger diuretics, and, in a glorious sunny room high up on the new cardiac floor at the hospital, with the kindest roommate a fellow patient ever had, Sam peed away seventeen pounds in ten days.

"No wonder he complained that he felt full and that it hurt him to walk," Dr. Wakely said. "Think how you'd feel carrying around a seventeen-pound bottle of water all day." Parker and I presumed from this that acid indigestion had not been Sam's complaint.

Dr. Wakely told us that he wanted Sam to stay in the hospital until he reached a sure dry weight and until the blood tests revealed a more normal state of affairs.

"It was confusing at the beginning," he explained, "because he only weighed one hundred and sixty-two pounds when he checked into the hospital. For his height he should be carrying that much weight anyway, and no one could possibly have suspected that so much of it was fluid. I'm afraid his heart just isn't pumping strongly enough to keep it off anymore, even with the stimulant he's been taking. We'll have to start him on something stronger."

There was absolutely no question of Sam's going right back to Kent. He would have to build back to activity very slowly and a step at a time.

School, however, was the last thing on Parker's mind and mine because, unlike the time Sam had gone into the hospital in August, the loss of fluid didn't seem to make him feel better at all. He submitted to the countless proddings and pokings of each day and to the indignities of all the tests without one word of complaint, but he was listless and withdrawn, while the migraines came relentlessly and the cough was continual.

"Cheer up, Sammy," Mr. Snow, his roommate, would say. "Tonight when the nurses go home we'll make buttered popcorn with lots of salt," and Sam would always smile. Poor Mr. Snow's diet was of an appalling blandness.

Mr. Snow left the hospital before Sam did, and, happy as we were for him, it was a bitter blow to have him replaced by a man who complained about being put in a room with a kid. "What's a kid doing on the cardiac floor anyway?" I heard him protest to a nurse in the hall outside the door of the room.

Sam himself never went into the hall at all. "I hate having people look at me," he said. "I get all the exercise I need going to the can."

Parker and I took Sam home from the hospital on October 8, but before we did we talked at length about his condition with Dr. Wakely in our old stamping grounds in the cardiac waiting room on the eighth floor.

"I'm not happy about him at all," Dr. Wakely said.

"Do you think it's about time to begin at least to research this heart transplant business?" Parker asked.

Doctor Wakely had told us in June, and Parker Vanamee had agreed, that Stanford University Medical Center in California was the only place in the entire world that he could recommend to us for Sam.

P.V. himself had said, "If you do ever have to go as far as a heart transplant, the only person to do it is Dr. Norman Shumway at Stanford or one of the people out there working on his team. Shumway started all the research on heart transplants, he's done it the right way, and he's the only person getting sound results. Barnard was working with him at Stanford, and he trotted off to South Africa with all Shumway's ideas to grab the fanfare, but in the medical world it's Shumway who gets the glory.

"You know," P.V. had finished, "when I was at Vanderbilt one time, I think Bill Scott told me he knew Shumway, and I'm not sure that Shumway isn't a Vanderbilt man himself. That's one nice thing about having a cousin who's important in the medical world, Beek. If the worst comes to the worst, you could always ask Bill Scott to write a letter to Shumway for you."

When Parker repeated the suggestion that morning, Dr. Wakely's eyes lit up. "That could certainly be a help," he said. "Why don't you go ahead and get in touch with Dr. Scott? I'll write Stanford myself in the meantime and get their opinion on where Sam would fit into their program."

The three of us set off to talk to Sam, and, exactly as we had in June after the catheterization, we ran into Dr. Hall. Parker told him that Dr. Wakely had offered to write Stanford for us, and, exactly as he had tossed off the very idea of a heart transplant then, Dr. Hall now scoffed at the idea of a letter to Shumway.

"They wouldn't even look at him," he exclaimed and explained to Parker and to me that there were four different and distinct stages of cardiac disease. "They won't even evaluate candidates for a heart transplant out there unless they're in Class Four — or end stage — heart failure. At least they'd have to be at the bottom of Class Three. Sam's still in Class One, barely going into Class Two."

Dr. Wakely didn't say anything, and Parker and I didn't either, but after we took Sam home, Parker went back to the office and wrote Bill Scott at Vanderbilt: "Please, if you know Shumway, will you write to him about Sam?"

What we took our cardiac patient home to was criminal. We were still at the Cape cottage, and after September one lives there in constant peril of frozen water pipes in the morning. In truth, we had no alternative because the new house, guaranteed to be finished in June, was only now nearing completion. The addition, housing a bedroom for Parker and me and a living room that could hold nine Pooles, still looked like a pipe dream to me.

"But it will be done for Christmas won't it, Mr. Bruce?" I'd asked the contractor brightly.

"I hope so," he'd answered, without the slightest hint of confidence in his voice.

I had gotten a downstairs bedroom ready for Sam at the new house while he was in the hospital. The movers had brought back our furniture from their warehouse, and I had shifted and sorted and unpacked enough belongings to make that one room look habitable, but Sam would have none of it.

He listened to me politely when I suggested that he could spend the days up there where it would be warmer and where he'd have Dottie and me for company, and he said maybe, but he stayed at the cottage. "I just don't want everyone up there looking at me and thinking I'm sick," he told me later by way of explanation.

The temperature in Maine plunges into the thirties almost every night after the first of October. The fall sun completely bypasses the front rooms of the cottage, shining — and then only late in the afternoon — on Sam and Charlie's bedroom and on a tiny little room off the upstairs bathroom that we use as a guest room. I moved Sam in up there, hoping that its smallness might hold the sun's warmth a little longer than his own huge room, but by nine o'clock at night it was Seward's Icebox along with everywhere else. We had bought a gas floor heater for the kitchen to supplement the one in the living-room window while Sam was in the hospital, but the cottage defied again, as it always had, the laws of physical science. In it, heat does not rise; it travels horizontally out through the walls of the building, and every morning at dawn Parker would tear to the bathroom to turn on the water faucets.

"We won," he'd exclaim, coming back to the bedroom. "They didn't freeze today," and we'd huddle on the edge of our bed, savoring the warmth of our coffee cups and steeling ourselves to exchange nightclothes for day clothes. The moment betwixt and between was exquisite in its agony.

At seven thirty, with Parker and Alix off to work and to school, I would repair to the new house to unpack and put away, leaving a note for Sam to call me when he woke up. At about ten thirty the phone at the new house would ring, and it would be Sam.

"Hi," he'd say glumly.

"I'll be right down and get your breakfast," I'd say. "Are you okay?"

He always said he didn't want any breakfast and that he was fine, but I always had to go down to see for myself. Invariably he would be wrapped in a down puff in the rocking chair in front of the gas heater in the living room. Hair soaking wet from his shower and straggling down over his eyes, he sat there slumped in the chair, doing nothing and close enough to the heater to ignite.

"Oh, God, Sam," I'd say, "you'll get a migraine from sitting there with all that hot air blowing on you. Won't you please come up to the other house? It's so awful down here." But he'd just shake his head.

"Maybe later," he'd say, and I'd go back to my chores at the new house, torn between hating to leave him alone and the urgency of getting him moved to a place with heat.

When Sam did talk, it was mostly about school. "I just want to go back to Kent," he'd protest every night. "I talked to the guys there on the phone today, and I'm missing so much I'll never get caught up. I had all this stuff planned for Blue Key too, and the kid who's doing it for me will never get it right."

But he accepted Dr. Wakely's word as law, and Dr. Wakely still said, "No, Sam. Not until we get things straightened out."

Dr. Wakely did think, however, that my idea to have Sam go to Waynflete, the day school in Portland where he'd gone before Kent, was a good idea. The headmaster of Waynflete himself was so sympathetic to Sam's problem that I could barely get out of his office with my dignity intact and the tears held back, and it was arranged that Sam would start classes there on Monday, October 18. The headmaster talked to Hart Perry at Kent, and between them a program was set up that would ensure Sam the number of credits he needed to graduate and would permit him to fit back into Kent courses when he was able to return to school.

Sam's first day at Waynflete was his last. He had an appointment with Dr. Wakely that same afternoon, and when I met him at the office he looked terrible. He barely protested when Dr. Wakely said, after he'd checked him over, "I think we'd better cut out the idea of school for now, Sam. I don't want you doing anything that strenuous."

"If I could sleep better at night," Sam said, "I know I'd get better, but I cough so much, and when I take the cough syrup it makes me throw up. I can't go to the can anymore either. I just never go to the bathroom at all."

Dr. Wakely gave him a prescription for pills for the cough instead of syrup and recommended bran and a laxative for his other complaint, and we went back for yet one more frigid night at the cottage.

Sam seemed relieved that he didn't have to go back to Waynflete. "There's something at Kent that doesn't mean the same unless you do the whole thing there," he said when we got home, "and I'm going to finish there. All I want is to go back," and after that, when I'd go down to the cottage to check on him during the day, one of the books he'd brought home from Kent would always be open on my desk next to the gas heater in the living room. Sam, however, would be wrapped in the down puff in front of the heater, with the rocking chair turned to face the television set.

"Did you get any reading done?" I'd ask.

And he always said, although I never quite knew what he meant, "I tried to, but it just isn't the same."

There were only sixteen days between the eighth, when Sam got out of the hospital, and the twenty-fifth, when he got into his bed at the new house. They might as well have been years. With every visit to Dr. Wakely's office, the row of pills on the bathroom shelf grew longer and longer, and I wrote to Tina that I couldn't understand how Sam's stomach could possibly feel well with all those compounds sloshing around in it. The only two bright spots in every day were at three thirty, when Alix got home from school for her routine tease, and at five thirty, when Pokie got home from the office.

"Didn't lose any weight at school today, did ya, Al?" Sam would say. "You oughta lend me a little of that rear, dear," and Alix would obligingly shriek "Mummeeeee!" just so he'd know he hadn't lost his touch.

Pokie religiously brought him the news of the day and, even better, the news of the night before from the bars, because there was no question by now of Sam's picking it up for himself.

On Thursday afternoon, October 21, it poured. I had distastefully picked my way down into the dank wetness of the cellar at the new house to put away some paints that the workmen had finished with, and I was surprised when I heard Sam calling me from the top of the stairs.

"Oh, great! You've come to visit," I exclaimed, starting up the stairs toward him.

"No," he said, "I'll come down. I don't want anyone else around."

There was a little chair with the back broken off it that I was using as a step stool, and he sat down heavily on that. He didn't say anything, though, for the longest time, and finally he put his head down and held it with his hands. I could see that he was trying not to cry, and I just stood in front of him trying not to myself.

It wasn't any use. He looked up at me with the tears pouring down his cheeks and said, "Oh, Mum, I don't think I can take it much more. Isn't there anything anyone can do? God, doesn't anyone know what to do? If I only knew — if just someone knew. I can't go on like this much more," and he put his head back down in his hands and wept.

I'd seen him cry briefly before, and sometimes I'd known that he had been crying, but all the bottled-up despair of the past months poured out that afternoon. His shoulders shook, and he was crying and coughing, and the damn rain was pouring through the ledge walls of the cellar, and I couldn't bear it anymore. I had to give him something to hope for; I didn't care what.

"Sam," I said, "there's a doctor in California who does all kinds of things with hearts, and we're waiting for a letter from him. Dr. Wakely's written him, and Daddy's asked Uncle Bill Scott to write him from Vanderbilt, and nothing's come yet, but it will. I promise you it will. Don't give up now because" — and I made myself smile at him — "because we might be on our way to California. I told you Daddy and I would take you anywhere in the world, and a doctor in California sure as heck beats one in Alaska at this time of year, doesn't it?"

That was the end of it. He didn't ask me anything more, and I still don't know what I would have said if he had.

On Monday, the twenty-fifth, the pipes froze at the cottage. The painters and plumbers and carpenters had finally withdrawn to the new addition, and we were going to move into the old part of the new house on Tuesday.

"This is crazy," I said to Sam on Monday when he got up. "I don't want you down here anymore. I want you to sleep up at the new house tonight," and he did.

That night, however, for some unexplained reason the main fuse at the new house blew, and when I got there Tuesday morning it was as cold as the cottage had ever been. There was no hot water for the shower that seemed to be Sam's only tonic, and I stood in the kitchen and swore at the top of my lungs.

When Sam woke up one morning the following week, he was terribly sick, but he did have an appointment to see Dr. Wakely at four that afternoon. He alternated all morning between vomiting and coughing attacks, and the mucus that came up now terrified me. It was no longer just streaked with dark stains; it was all bright red with blood, and I could only think, as I pressed a wet washcloth to his forehead or cracked ice for him to suck on, Oh, thank God for the appointment!

At two I turned my post over to Dottie and went to market, but when I came back Dottie told me that Parker had called and that he had canceled Sam's appointment for that afternoon. It was to be the next day at the same time.

"How could you?" I shrieked over the phone at poor Parker. "Here's Sam so sick he can't stand up and you've canceled the appointment. Dr. Wakely has got to see him today!"

Sometimes I wonder why Parker puts up with me, but instead of telling me how awful I was he only said, "I'm sorry; I didn't know. Dr. Wakely has something he wants to talk to us about, and he wanted a little more time to check it out. He called me here at the office, but I'll call him right back and tell him Sam needs to see him today."

Sam felt a little better when we got to Dr. Wakely's office, and I felt a little foolish about my histrionics. We had barely sat down to wait when the receptionist came over to me and said, "Mrs. Poole, you have a phone call."

I was surprised, because only Dottie and Parker knew where I was, and I couldn't imagine why either of them would be calling me at the doctor's office. It was even more bewildering to be led past the phone on the receptionist's desk through a maze of corridors into what appeared to be a laboratory.

"Where's the phone?" I asked.

"It's really not a call, Mrs. Poole," the receptionist explained. "It's Dr. Wakely. He wants to talk to you."

"But isn't he here at the office?" I asked, totally confused.

"He's in his own office," she explained deliberately. "He doesn't want Sam to hear."

They handed me a telephone, pushed a button, and indeed I heard Dr. Wakely's voice.

"I've heard from Stanford," he said, and he sounded as excited and delighted as if the good news were for his own child. "They want to see Sam. I've told Mr. Poole, and he should be here any minute now, but I wanted to tell you before we talk to Sam that I don't think the heart transplant should be mentioned today. I don't think Sam should be told yet."

Dumbfounded, I hung up. How could we not tell him? "What will I say to Sam?" I asked a technician who was in the room; the receptionist had departed. "Who will I say was on the phone?"

"Make up something," she said.

I'm a rotten liar, which keeps me more honest than I ever intend to be. I blush and I squirm and I explain too much. "I had to talk to Dottie," I said to Sam, and dumb as it sounds, I had. I had dialed our number, and when she said hello I had said, "Hello, Dottie, I'll explain later," and hung up.

"I thought she called you," Sam protested, but before I had to continue weaving my tangled web, Parker appeared, and the three of us went into Dr. Wakely's office.

He checked Sam over in the examining room and then rejoined us with Sam in the office. "I had a call from a Doctor John Schroeder at Stanford University today, Sam," he started out, "and I had a long talk with him about you. He's very interested in your case. I'd written him about you, and your uncle at Vanderbilt has evidently written to Stanford too. They'd like you to come out to California to take a look at you."

"What for?" Sam asked. "Is there anything they could do?"

"Well, Sam," Parker said, "there might be some kind of an operation that could help you, and —"

I couldn't stand it anymore. I sat there in my chair and looked at Sam and remembered that awful day in the cellar when he'd sat on the broken chair and cried. I kept hearing him saying, "If I only knew — if just someone knew," and I blurted out the whole thing.

"Sam, you know you're awfully sick," I said, "and the only way you can keep from dying is to have a heart transplant. There isn't any other alternative."

I'd done it. I'd been the hatchet man, and I sat there in my chair, waiting in terror for everyone to say, "How could you say such a thing? You've ruined everything!" and for Sam to break down.

He didn't. He sat up straight in his chair and demanded, "Why didn't somebody tell me before? I just wanted to know that there was something they could do. That's great!"

Parker reached over and put his hand on Sam's knee, Dr. Wakely positively beamed, and the hatchet man started shaking all over.

Chapter Six

I don't think I said another word during the whole time the three of us sat in Dr. Wakely's office that Monday afternoon. I couldn't take my eyes off Sam. He leaned forward eagerly in his chair, and suddenly he was a seventeen-year-old boy again who knows, as all seventeen-year-old boys know, that of course there is something somebody can do about everything. It hurt him too much to tie his shoes anymore, but even his feet in the old Adidas with the dangling laces didn't look so wilted to me.

"What does it involve?" he asked Dr. Wakely. "You know, what are the things I gotta do?"

Dr. Wakely just shook his head. "Sam," he said, "there's nobody like you!" and the moment of shock was over for us all.

I have no idea how long our appointment lasted, but every minute of it was ours. If Dr. Wakely had a dozen patients waiting outside his office that afternoon, he gave no indication of it.

He started off with a review of what had happened in the

nine months since January when Sam's heart condition had been discovered. Dr. Owens at Massachusetts General, he reminded us, had noted, in his letter written in June, a slight increase in the size of the heart, but on the whole Sam had managed to get along fairly well until August, when Dr. Mansfield had put him in the hospital with the so-called full feeling. At that time, even before diuretics and heart stimulants were started, Sam's body had managed to eliminate the fluid that was beginning to build up. He was taking mild dosages of both when he became Dr. Wakely's patient two weeks later, just before he went back to Kent. It had been impossible then to detect the presence of any fluid at all, even though in all probability Sam had begun once again to accumulate it. It was the two weeks at Kent, trying to lead a normal life, that proved, of course, that his heart simply couldn't supply enough blood to his organs for them to function properly and to dispel the fluids.

"When we got you back into the hospital, Sam," he said, "we realized that you were going into congestive heart failure, but no one thought it was going to come on so suddenly or progress so quickly. Here it is only two-and-a-half weeks since you left the hospital, and things have gotten considerably worse. It really is time we did something."

It was like coming out of an endless tunnel. In March after Dr. Hall had told us that the heart would never get better, I had said to Sam, "We're all in this together," but since June we hadn't been. We had hidden from him the awful conclusions established by the catheterization. Even now I guess it was the right thing to do. We couldn't have said that summer, "Well, Sam, old boy, you're going to die sometime in the next few years unless you have a transplant." If it happened all over again, I still couldn't say that. There had to be a time to say it, and the time was that afternoon in Dr. Wakely's office when suddenly a heart transplant was a reality, not a vague future dread, and I looked at Parker and smiled.

You have to know Parker a long time to know what he's thinking. "The great stone face," I used to call him when we first got engaged, but over the years I've noticed that his brown eyes crinkle just a little at the edges when he's pleased and his mouth goes straight. When he's upset his lower lip goes in slightly and twists. It had been in and twisting a lot that summer, but not that afternoon. I knew he was thinking, Thank God, now we're telling it like it is, and I knew that he felt as I did that, for the first time since January, we had a chance.

Sam must have felt that way too. Dr. Wakely hadn't needed to tell him how sick he was or that something had to be done, and there was no shock or dismay on his face at all — just that wonderful look of eagerness I hadn't seen for so long.

"So when do I go to California?" he asked, and we settled back in our chairs to listen to Dr. Wakely telling us how one went about getting a heart transplant. A coach giving his team the Saturday game plan could not have commanded more rapt attention.

Dr. Schroeder, explained Dr. Wakely, was the cardiologist on Dr. Shumway's team who provided the link between Stanford and prospective transplants. He had discussed with Dr. Wakely the prerequisites for getting accepted into the heart transplant program, and one of them had to be accomplished before a trip to California could even be contemplated. We three — Sam, Parker, and I — must first agree to see a psychiatrist in Portland to determine whether we were strong enough to undergo what Dr. Wakely said could only be described as a real ordeal.

I was listening so intently that it wasn't till I heard Sam say, "You mean we can't go right away? How long will the psychiatrist thing take?" and heard the disappointment in his voice that I turned to look at him and say that his new-found enthusiasm had faded.

Dr. Wakely looked at Sam directly. "Not too long, Sam," he said, "but you've got to understand that getting a new heart is going to be a long, drawn-out process from start to finish. There's no use leaping into this until you know exactly what's expected of you and whether you want to commit yourself to it."

He looked at Parker and me then and added, "I'm sure I don't have to tell you that it's an expensive process as well, but you might not realize how much of a commitment it will be for the two of you. A heart transplant has to be a team effort all the way — and that doesn't mean just Dr. Shumway's team at Stanford, either. It means you, the Poole family, too." We would have to be willing to move to Palo Alto, where Stanford is located, for an extended period of time, we would have to have enough money to set up headquarters there and to pay for any hospitalization for Sam until his heart arrived, and we would have to pledge ourselves to stick with him every inch of the way.

"They've discovered out there that transplant recipients need family support during every phase of the transplant process. No one could be expected to endure it alone."

Dr. Wakely smiled at us. "I told Dr. Schroeder I didn't think he had to worry about you on that score, but you have to understand that it can take up to three months just to find a heart that would properly match with Sam's blood type and tissues. The better the heart is suited to him, the better are his chances of avoiding a massive rejection. You know," he said — and he couldn't have put it better — "they don't just pick a heart off the shelf."

We all laughed at that, even Sam. "I don't care where they get it from or how long it takes, just as long as we're waiting for something," he said, and Dr. Wakely smiled again.

"I know, Sam, but I want you to understand just what's involved in this. After you actually get your heart, one of your parents will have to stay in California to be with you while you're in the hospital, and that's a long time too. Even after you're out of the hospital you'll have to stay in the Stanford area until Dr. Shumway's team decides you can come home to Maine, and of course," he said, turning to Parker, "you or Mrs. Poole will have to be with him for that time as well.

"It's a lot of time and a lot of money any way you look at it," Dr. Wakely went on. "A government grant pays for the operation itself and for the recuperative care in the hospital afterward, but, as I said, you would have to cover all prior hospitalization costs until that time came. When you add on your living expenses and his, it's a major financial commitment." He had told Dr. Schroeder, he said, that he knew we would be able to work out some way to handle the financial end and that he was sure that going to a psychiatrist wouldn't bother us.

"It's an absolute must," he said, "before you can even begin to sort out any other matters. Evidently some potential candidates have gotten out there in the past, and either they or their families simply haven't been able to get through the whole course. Do you happen to have a psychiatrist you'd feel comfortable with, or do you know of one you'd like to see?"

In our family no one has ever needed a psychiatrist to diagnose what is wrong with him or her; there are ten people standing daily, ready in line, to convey that message. Sam and Parker and I mutely shook our heads.

Dr. Wakely laughed. "Well, I do," he said. "I know quite a few, but the man I'd like you to see, and the man I'd have one of my own kids go to, is Dr. Frederick Bushman. I know you'll like him and be able to talk to him, and I think he's even worked with a prospective heart transplant before, when they were doing the operation in New York. I'll call him and see if he can talk to the three of you.

"You know, Sam," he said, "this isn't a decision you have to make today. There's going to be a lot of pain involved; truly, 'ordeal' is the only word to describe it. The operation itself, transferring the heart into your body, is a relatively simple one, but the aftermath can be very unpleasant, and, worst of all, there are no guarantees that the whole thing will work. Rejection and disease will become your natural enemies."

Dr. Wakely carefully explained the process of rejection to us. The body does not care for foreign matter of any kind, and the white cells in the blood work endlessly to repel all boarders. Germs, splinters, or new hearts — they're all one and the same to the white cells. To counteract their opposition and to force the body to accept a transplanted organ, the white cells must be kept suppressed with drugs, which in turn leaves the body with no defense mechanism against disease. What's more, the drugs themselves can often produce miserable and hazardous side effects.

"There are antirejection shots you'll have to have, Sam,"

Dr. Wakely finished, "that, according to Stanford, are unbelievably painful; and should you survive the operation itself, and all the rejections and all the diseases, and suffer through all the pain, you still have to remember that a heart transplant is not a cure. You are going to have to take those drugs with all their unpleasant side effects for the rest of your life, and you're going to be tied to doctors and hospitals for the rest of your life too. You've really got to think the whole thing over very carefully."

And Sam said quietly, in an absolutely matter-of-fact voice, "I know, Dr. Wakely, I will. But when you look at the alternatives, what are they?"

If someone had told me that I was going to die unless I was willing to endure terrible suffering and, having endured it, might still quite possibly die, I know I couldn't have asked that question the way Sam did. To begin with, I know I would have been crying too hard to speak.

I think Dr. Wakely was impressed too, because he cleared his throat twice before he said to Parker that Dr. Schroeder would like him to call Lois Christopherson, the social-service worker in charge of the heart transplant program at Stanford, as soon as possible. "She can fill you in on all the details of what will happen if Sam should decide to go through with this and will make arrangements for an evaluation of his condition at Stanford," he said.

He gave Parker her name and her number and called in a new prescription for Sam at our drugstore, and we left.

When we got outside, Sam turned to me and said, "Mum, I'd like to drive home myself. You go with Dad. I want to go alone." And even though we stopped at the drugstore for the prescription, we got home long before he did.

Being alone seemed almost the only visible dignity he had left, and I tried not to worry when he went off in the car by himself, but I couldn't help feeling relieved when he appeared in the kitchen in about twenty-five minutes. I knew, looking at him, that he had been crying, but all he said was, "Are you going to call that lady tonight, Dad?"

"I'd like to," Parker said, "if you want me to."

There was no hesitation. "Hell, yes," he said. "Let's get going; I just thought on the way home — now I'll be able to say 'I Left My Heart in San Francisco' is my theme song."

Parker talked to Lois Christopherson at about eight o'clock Maine time that night, after we finally organized the three-hour time difference between East and West in our minds. At the best of times, nothing is more frustrating than listening to only one end of an important phone call. That night it was unendurable. When we remodeled the kitchen, the architect had placed an island of shelves in the middle of the floor, and Sam sat in a chair at the kitchen table on one side of it while Parker stood at the telephone on the other side. I fumbled my way around the island, trying to clean up from supper as if everything were quite normal and biting my lip to keep from demanding of Parker, "What did she say?" when I was on his side of the island, and of Sam, "What do you think she said?" when I was on his. Finally I heard Parker say, "But he's right here in the kitchen with us."

There was a pause, and then Parker burst out laughing. Sam and I waited impatiently for the conversation to end, and finally he said, "Well, he says his theme song is going to be 'I Left My Heart in San Francisco,' " and hung up.

Parker's face at that moment was anything but impassive. "She couldn't believe you knew about it, Sam," he exulted. "She asked me how we were planning to break the news about the transplant to you, and when I told you you were right here with us, she couldn't believe it. That's what got me laughing. I guess she thinks you must be a pretty tough fella."

He told us what else she had said. Should we decide to go to Stanford and if Sam were judged to be a suitable candidate for a new heart after a five- to ten-day evaluation of his condition at the hospital there, he would then be on the official list to wait for a heart. If he were accepted as a candidate, one of three things could happen. He might be considered sick enough to warrant hospitalization at Stanford during the wait, he might be released from the hospital to wait in the Stanford area, or, undreamed-of hope, he might be considered well enough to return home until a suitable heart was found for him.

In any case but the last, Parker said, we would have to make living arrangements for ourselves in the Stanford area. There were no facilities provided for future transplant patients or their families. The waiting time could last from a day to three months, and there was a guaranteed two- to three-month stay in the hospital after the new heart was implanted. "Add on another two to three months that have to be spent near Stanford after a transplant is released from the hospital," Parker said, "and she says you're looking at anywhere from six to nine months."

My arithmetic is faulty at best, and while I laboriously transferred us from November to August on my fingers, I heard Parker telling Sam that Lois, as she had instructed him to call her, wanted us to think things over and to call her back when we had come to a definite decision.

"Well, Sammy," Parker said, "what do you think?"

Sam had been sitting in his usual position hunched over the table, and he didn't say anything for a second or two. Then he stood up and looked squarely at Parker and said, "I think we gotta go. I thought about it coming home from

Dr. Wakely's; I stopped the car and I just thought. At first it made me mad, like, you know, Geez, why me? Out of everybody, why me? — but it *is* me, Dad, and we know how bad it is, and we know what we can do about it now, so I guess we gotta go."

It was the longest speech I'd heard him make since he'd been sick, and afterward the three of us sat together and talked in the kitchen and planned. It was wonderful just to be able to plan again.

That night when Parker and I got into the miserable isolation of the twin beds in the guest room where we had been forced to take up quarters until our new room was finished, Parker said, "You know what I was thinking in Dr. Wakely's office this afternoon? I was thinking how great it was that we were telling it to Sammy like it is, and that everything is out in the open now."

"I knew you were," I said with considerable satisfaction.

I spent the whole next day wondering how you went to live in California, and how you coped with a twelve-year-old while you were gone, but there was never a question in my mind that we were going. The only thing that I found myself surprised at was that only a month ago when Sam was in the hospital a heart transplant had been somewhere in the dark dim future, and suddenly it wasn't.

When Parker came home that night, he called Lois Christopherson at Stanford again and said, "We're coming." She didn't even say that we would have to wait for the outcome of the talks with the Portland psychiatrist, which were to start on November 8; she said we could come anytime after November 21, and what was Sam's blood type?

None of us knew, but Parker said, "I'll call the doctor and let you know tomorrow," while I ran off to my desk for my trusty Episcopalian church calendar, which confuses life by ignoring things like Washington's Birthday and the Fourth of July but happily includes Thanksgiving among its Saint's Days and Feasts.

Parker looked at it for a second and then he said, "Why don't we come out on Monday, the twenty-ninth? We'll have almost the whole family home for Thanksgiving, and I think Sam would like to see everyone before we leave. We'll be out the next Monday."

It developed the next day that, with all the hundreds of vials of blood that had been drawn from Sam since January, no one had any idea of what his blood type was. It seemed bizarre, but it was an easily correctable matter. By five o'clock that afternoon we had learned that he was, in fact, Type O Negative, and Parker had set the wheels in motion for our new lives.

He looked like the cat that ate the canary when he came home that night. "Stick with me, kid," he said to Sam, "and you'll go first-class," and he plunked down three round-trip tickets to San Francisco on the kitchen table in front of Sam. When we looked at them, there was no question that when Parker Poole said first-class, he meant first-class.

"My God," I said, "I don't believe it. Pooles don't travel first-class."

"They do when they're having heart transplants," Parker said. "Sam likes to be comfortable, don't you, Sammy? And I want to watch him be comfortable."

It was done. In twenty-six days we would be living in California, and all Parker and I had left to sort out were the children, the dog, the house, Christmas, and that bête noire of anyone who has six children — money.

We didn't talk about such minor matters that night with

Sam there, but, as if by signed agreement, we both got up the next morning at four and went to the kitchen. There was no companionable edge-of-the-bed sitting in the guest room. The old pine beds were so high that my feet didn't even touch the floor, so we had our coffee sitting in two rocking chairs in front of the Franklin stove in the kitchen.

"And on the porch veranda sat Silas and Miranda," I would croak at Parker every morning.

"Not today," he said, as I started off that morning. "We've got a lot to plan out."

By six forty-five we had conquered every obstacle but one. Alix, Moriah, and the house would be in Dottie's charge when we took Sam to California. Malcolm was being discharged from the Coast Guard in December, and he and Ruthie, who had recently bought a house near Portland, were planning to live in ours until their own was ready anyway. They could take over, with Dottie coming by the day, until one of us could get back from California.

Pokie had rented a house two miles away for the winter with some friends, Charlie was at Trinity, and Tina was in England. That covered children, house, and dog.

Planning for Christmas took the longest, because the logistics were confusing. After Sam's evaluation, if he were not judged well enough to wait for his heart at home, we would take an apartment in Palo Alto. Leaving Parker with Sam, I would return home to get things ready for Christmas, going back to our western outpost in time for Parker to come back to see the other children before Christmas. We were agreed that on Christmas Eve he would return to California so that we could both be with Sam on Christmas Day. Tina was coming back from England for the holidays, and there was no question in our minds that she and Ruthie, with a little precooking help from Dottie and advice from Rozzie, could easily handle the East Coast Christmas. After that, Parker and I would alternate three-week stints of duty on one coast or the other.

"Money?" I asked nervously. "What will we do about money? Mother's and Daddy's estates aren't settled, and we've got all the bills for the new house coming in. Where are we going to get the money?"

Parker is used to debt. When he sold our old house in Portland in 1975, he made a great announcement to the children. "For the first time since I married your mother," he had solemnly stated, "I am out of debt. I'll probably be right back in tomorrow, but not tonight," and he had therewith handed each of them a check for two hundred dollars.

"We share the good times," he had said, "and we share the bad," and that was all I could think of that morning when I brought up the problem of finances.

"Don't worry," Parker said. "We're going to California and we're going to do this thing for Sam regardless of what it's going to cost, so let's not waste time and energy on that. We coped with Pokie's operations, and we'll cope with this thing. After all, I can always go back into debt again. God knows I've been that route before, and the company insurance will help too."

The only thing we couldn't sort out before breakfast that morning was Dottie's husband, Don Libby. He worked for Parker's company, and although Parker and I were devoted to him, and although he had always stayed with Dottie at our house when we were away, Local 340 of the Teamsters Union was on strike at the Shurtleff Company. It had been an awkward month for all four of us. "It will be hard for Don staying here," Parker said. "The other guys on the wharf are going to give him an awfully hard time if they find out he's living in management's house."

By 9 A.M. on Thursday, even that obstacle was gone. "Don and I have already talked about it," Dottie told me. "We both agree that Sam comes ahead of everything else." What came to replace dilemmas of the future was an immediate one. Sam came downstairs about ten thirty. I had heard him coughing and gagging through his hour shower and had just started cracking his morning supply of the ice that had become breakfast, lunch, and dinner for him. Aside from a grilled cheese sandwich from time to time and Jell-O, he ate nothing else at all.

"Are you going to the trustees' meeting at Kent tomorrow?" he demanded.

"Good heavens, no," I said. "Kent will understand. I couldn't bear to go there with you here sick."

"I want to go with you," he said. "I want to get my stereo and I want to say good-bye to my friends. I want to tell them myself."

I told Dr. Wakely, and he simply said, "He probably shouldn't, but I think it's important that he go," and so we went.

Sam insisted on driving part of the way, and the car wove and wobbled along the highway with no respect at all for lanes. It poured to boot, and, when the windshield wipers broke, he got livid because I wouldn't let him stand outside in the rain to fiddle with them. I got out myself and inadvertently shut his arm in the car door when he reached out to show me what to do. Only after we drove across the steel bridge that spans the Housatonic River, separating the school from the town of Kent, did the miseries of the past five hours seem worthwhile. Hart Perry must have told Sam's friends that he was coming, because a bunch of boys were lounging on the grass at the head of the school driveway.

"There he is!" someone yelled, spotting our Maine license plate, and someone else yelled, "It's the man, himself!" and our car was surrounded by a raucous escort all the way to the parking lot. No sooner had Sam stopped the car than the blue-jeaned, sneakered throng had his door open, and he made what for him was almost a leap into its midst.

"Hey there, Benny. What's up, you guys? You keepin' your noses clean without me?" I could hear his voice all the way across the parking lot, but I couldn't distinguish his departing back in the mob that engulfed him, as he headed toward his old dorm to spend the night.

I stayed with the Perrys, and, although I must have gone to the trustees' meeting, I can't remember anything about it. I do remember forcing myself not to ask Hart to have one of the prefects check on Sam before we went to bed, but to my relief he did it himself.

"Sam's having a ball," he said, but the next morning I was still in my nightgown in Hart's study, which converts to a guest room at night, when I heard the most ghastly retchings and coughings. I rushed over to the window and saw Sam staggering up the steep hill which is topped by the Perrys' house. Fran must have heard him too, and I met her at the front door — "diphaneous" (as the children call "diaphanous") nightgown and all.

Sam was all bent over, clutching his sides and coughing. "I gotta get to the can," he groaned and rushed past us into the bathroom.

We helped him into the car twenty minutes later. Hart had offered to drive home with me, and I was frightened to go alone, but I couldn't let him do it.

"No," I said, "it'll be fine," but of course it wasn't. There wasn't any question of Sam's driving. He lay far in the corner of the front seat with his head thrown back, and the most dreadful noises kept coming out of his throat. He was sweating all over, even though it was a cold morning, and I drove, but I don't know how. Once I stopped at a restaurant to get him some cracked ice and found I was terrified at leaving him alone in the car.

"Hurry," I pleaded with the girl at the counter. "I'll pay you for the ice, but please hurry."

Just after the first exit of the Maine Turnpike, the noise stopped. Oh, God, I said to myself, he's died. I looked over at him, and there was no sign of his being alive at all. There was no noise, there was no breathing; his mouth was open and his eyes were shut.

Oh, God, I thought, how do you get off a turnpike with someone who's dead in the car?

By the time we were getting near the next exit, I had decided how you did it. When you stopped at the tollbooth, you said, "Get me an ambulance!" But just then the gasping started again. Out of the corner of my eye, I could see his chest pounding crazily, and for some peculiar reason I didn't stop at that exit at all. I just kept going until we reached our own, paid the toll as if nothing were wrong, and drove home. By the time we got to the Cape, the gasping and the pounding had stopped.

He never got out of bed until Sunday morning. I kept going to his door to peek in and see if he was all right, and every time he was lying motionless, but wide awake. "Are you okay?" I'd ask, and he'd answer in a dead, hollow voice that frightened me, "Oh, I'm so tired." It was well after midnight when the words became sobs, and I went over to him then and sat on the edge of the bed, rubbing his shoulder.

"Oh, darling, it was all my fault," I said after a minute or two. "I should never have let you go," but he pulled impatiently away from me when I said that and lifted his head off the pillow.

"I had to go," he said fiercely. "Don't you understand? I had to say good-bye to my friends."

I couldn't believe my eyes when he got up on Sunday morning. He seemed happier than he'd been in ages, and it was hard to believe that the trip home and the anguish of the night before had been anything more than a nightmare. "Let's have a picnic at the Tea House with Aunt Roz and Uncle Bill," he said, and we did. He invited Freddie and another friend. Although it was a beautiful day, it was too cold even to consider sitting outside, so we all huddled around the little fireplace inside, and Uncle Bill, who hadn't seen Sam since the plans for California had come up, flung his arms around him when he got there.

"My boy," he exclaimed, "you must write a book! You will make the family fortune!" and even though Sam insisted, "Gawd, Uncle Bill, who cares about a fortune? I'd be satisfied if I could smoke a butt or party again," the rest of us decided that Bill was right.

"Except," Freddie dismally pointed out, "there wouldn't be any sex in it. You gotta have sex, Sam, to sell a book, but you'll be too busy to find any. We'll have to collaborate; you write about getting the heart, and I'll fill in the sexy parts."

It was such a grand day. I felt happier about Sam after that picnic at the Tea House than I had since the Tea House dance, four months before, when he'd partied himself into sickness on the same site.

"Sometimes I think he must be the bravest seventeen-year-old boy alive to be as good-natured as he is through all this mess," I wrote to Tina, and I added, "As good-natured as he *was*, that is, for today I wrecked the needle on his stereo cleaning it, and, my, was he mad — and I don't blame him."

That information came at the end of a letter written to her on November 8, the day after the picnic, from the psychiatrist's waiting room.

"My dearest elderly ugly daughter," I wrote. "You will never believe where Sam and I are sitting — in a psychiatrist's waiting room . . . about to be advised, I'm sure, that we are quite mad. Having been here for five minutes, it appears to be like any doctor's office — no straitjackets, couches, or screaming patients — and, oh, joy, even ashtrays. I can hardly wait till Dad arrives for our appointment in an hour. Can you envision him telling all to a psychiatrist? You know he won't, and the psychiatrist will start telling Dad his own problems, and at the end of the hour Dad will tell the psychiatrist to 'Shape up.' "

And a little later on, I wrote her: "Sam has just gone off with Dr. Bushman, who is not at all as I imagined him. He is Brooks Brothers from neck to waist and L. L. Bean below. On top (of the neck, that is), he looks rather like Malcolm or Charlie, which is comforting."

And even later, at the end of twelve pages: "You will be bored reading this, but it surely has made the time fly writing it. Psychiatrists are just like every other doctor: they make you wait!"

Sam went home after his time with Dr. Bushman was up. Parker had come for our appointment by then, and it was even more comforting to find that there were no couches in Dr. Bushman's inner office either. He sat at his desk and looked directly at me.

"Mrs. Poole," he said, "how do you feel about all this?"

"Awful," I said. "How else could I possibly feel?"

It had seemed the only reasonable thing to say, but then he asked, "And how do you feel about Sam's having a heart transplant? By now you know all the dangers and the pain that will be involved for him if he should have one."

"But what other choice do we have?" I asked. "They've told us it's his only hope."

"That's true," he said, "but there are a lot of people who would still rather not go through with it."

"But he'd die," I protested. "We can't just let him die."

Dr. Bushman never asked me any more questions about my feelings after that, and he never asked Parker anything at all. I think he looked at him and at his face and knew that if there was a weak link anywhere in the chain to keep Sam alive, it wasn't Parker.

After that, he was immeasurably helpful and dear. He had indeed worked with a man who was a candidate for a heart transplant in New York several years earlier, and he went over again with us the many unpleasant aspects of the entire procedure.

"Some people," he said, "actually would rather die than go through such agony, and many families don't want someone they love to have to go through it either. I want you to know that what I report from my meetings with you and with Sam won't influence in any way Stanford's decision to accept him, but it can perhaps save you from trying to do something you might decide you can't face.

"You must always remember that you will be going down two roads at once. On both roads you will meet the perils of such a procedure: rejection, disease, and always pain. At the end of one road, though, will be Sam alive, and at the end of the other he will be dead. The odds are about equal for both. If you decide to go through with the transplant, you must realize that you are always on both roads and accept their outcome without any feelings of guilt or remorse."

"Dr. Bushman," I said, "my brother died when he was born and my sister died when she was seven. Mother always told me that the agony for her forever was not knowing what they would have been like when they grew up. We have to give Sam this chance whatever happens; he wants to live. If he stays here, he would just die."

"Yes, he would," Dr. Bushman said quietly. "He would die, and you would have to watch him."

That was as metaphysical as we got. Parker hates to waste time on foregone conclusions. We were going to California, we had three round-trip first-class tickets to take us there, and, like the money problem, it was foolish to debate. He started asking Dr. Bushman entirely unpsychiatric questions about heart transplants: Who were the donors? Young males usually. How was the heart sustained during its transferral from one body to another? It was kept from degeneration in a solution. How bad could rejections be? Bad enough to make the new heart totally useless. Were the drugs used to fight rejection as painful and hazardous as we had been led to believe? Yes.

Dr. Bushman didn't seem to object to Parker's practical approach at all. He told us that he would like to meet with Sam another time, and with us again too, and as we were leaving he said, "I enjoyed talking to Sam. He's really quite mature for his age, and it's very good that he seems to feel so close to you. He says he loves you both very much. I think he is very courageous."

Sam was lying down on the tired old sofa in the

playroom behind the kitchen when we got home, and he looked just as faded and worn as it did. All the turntables, speakers, tape decks, and wires of his beloved stereo surrounded him as usual, but for once they were silent.

"Did you like Dr. Bushman?" we asked him.

"Yeah, he was okay," he said, "but all those questions and just going over everything made me so tired. Mum," he finished, "don't tell anybody I went, will you?"

The next morning I looked in the mirror and, selfish to the core, announced to Parker that I was going to New York. "I can cope with almost anything," I stated flatly, "but I cannot cope with a heart transplant without a haircut."

I took advantage of the fact that November 11 was a holiday in Maine in 1976 but not in New York, and, with Parker at home for the day, I left Sam in his charge that Thursday morning and set off. I returned to a sorry sight on Friday night. Sam had woken up with a migraine after I left — the worst one, he told Parker, that he had ever had. Parker had heard him in the bathroom and found him throwing up, shaking and covered with sweat. It had gone on all that day and all that night, and on Friday Parker had taken him to Dr. Wakely's office.

It was all from the headache, Dr. Wakely had assured him, but Parker told me when I got home that he was beginning to wonder how many of those sessions Sam could endure before his heart just gave out.

"He threw up in the trash pail in the car on the way home," Parker told me, "and the only time I saw him smile the whole two days was after he'd finished. He looked over at me and said, 'Pretty good, Dad, huh? I hit the bucket.' I could have cried."

We began to wonder after that if waiting to go to Stanford until Thanksgiving was over had been a terrible mistake. Taking each day at a time is a way of life I detest, but it became somehow the only way to survive. I tried to set up little schedules for myself — all within the house and between migraines — based on life as usual. I washed the woodwork in the kitchen on Mondays, and I cleaned the stove on Tuesdays, which, as I wrote to Tina, "would bore anyone but a mother, whom it makes happy and to whom it gives assurance that life will go on."

I wondered daily at my good fortune in having Parker for a husband and wrote Tina in the same letter that "my biggest recommendation to you is that you marry a man as unselfish as your father, for it is he who makes all things possible. Strikes, disasters, daily problems he finds the strength to tackle and cope with in such an inspired manner that how can I do less? If I am also forced to admit that he can be G. D. bossy (he in turn says I am, as we know too), he's not a bad deal for any of us. I do admire my taste of twenty-six years ago."

The idea of Sam's writing a book had captured Parker's fancy. "I'll be your agent, Sam," he had declared coming back from the Tea House picnic. "A straight ten percent and you can keep the rest." The idea evidently captured Sam's fancy too. He had started a journal the next day, on the eighth of November, the morning of our appointments with Dr. Bushman. He had been unable to write after the migraine came on the eleventh, but he'd brought it up to date on the fifteenth.

If Parker was to be the agent, I was evidently, with nothing to recommend me but a college English major, to be the editor. At night Sam would say, "Read this, Mum. Does it sound okay?'' and I would try hard to read it intellectually and to judge it academically. It was hard to do when there were excerpts like these:

Nov. 8, 1976 — Monday
  Today is a very significant day. I go to see Dr. Bushman. I am still tired from my escapade to Kent, but, God, am I glad I went. Those people mean a lot to me. As I told one friend — no matter how much anybody says they hate the place, if they ever had any friends there, they're full of shit.

  Dr. Bushman was O.K. . . . The idea of a shrink is worse than the real thing.

Nov. 9 — Tuesday
  . . . Fred came out today and gave me an album and a book from his parents. These people, I think, mean more to me than anybody with the exception of my parents and family, that is, Dot. They have a lot of love in them. Fred especially. If anything happened to me, I think he would know. I love him and his family and would do the same for him.

Nov. 10 — Wednesday
  . . . I just want to be able to live normally. It snowed today which made me feel good. I don't know why.
  We received a folder from Stanford . . . just procedures, but anything is progress.

November 11–14 (I am writing this the fifteenth)
  These four days have been recovery days. On Thursday I woke up and from the first I did not feel right. . . . The pain is worse and more constant than any pain I have had. . . . Thank God my father was here. . . .

Friday
  I feel physically drained; the headache is going down. My muscles

ache and throb — my neck and arms especially. Jell-O seems to be the only thing I can keep down.

Charlie came home . . . today. I'm glad. It is good to see him. I always tried to be as good as he was at Kent with crew and all. I'm glad and sorry I could never continue with crew. I feel very close to Charlie. We have always been, I think. I'm very glad it was me and not him who got sick. It would be unfair to him. . . . I am somehow the same without sports, but I couldn't — and I'm sure no one else could — stand to see Charlie idle.

Dottie nursed me all day. . . .

Saturday
Mum came home last night. I'm glad she's back. She went to New York City. She needs it every once in a while.

November 15 — Monday
I woke up very aggravated today. I had some weird dreams. In one of them someone told me I could not have the operation and I just remember something about saying, "I don't want to die." I just feel so useless.

November 16 — Tuesday
I received a package from Kent. It was the game ball from the Hotchkiss game. I can't explain how I felt. In a way I wished they had not sent it and in a way I'm glad. The people down there are super.

Later I got the full feeling and

That "and" was the end of the book.

The Hotchkiss game football had indeed come that morning. To a Kent student a win over Loomis or Taft is a good thing, but to defeat "the Kissies" is a glorious triumph, and even I realized that the football in Sam's package was not just a football. On it was inscribed darkly, in black Magic Marker: KENT — 23, HOTCHKISS — 6; and above that it said: FOR ANOTHER WINNER — SAM. The entire remaining area of the ball was covered with the signatures of all the players and the coach.

"Geez, they didn't have to do that," said old Number 71, and I took the ball and, turning my back to him, put it on the mantelpiece over the Franklin stove so that neither of us would have to see the other cry. When Parker saw it that night, he got very busy taking ice out of the refrigerator and feeding the dog with his back to us.

We lived in limbo for the remaining thirteen days before we went to Stanford, and sometimes it was hard to believe that, with luck, heaven could be equally as attainable as hell.

My moods fluctuated wildly. When I thought of Dr. Wakely's delight when we'd told him that we were going to go to Stanford, I knew that things were going to be fine. We were in his office, and he'd smiled at us and said, "I'm so pleased. What's a heart, after all? It's just an old pump, and if Sam's is all worn out, it's high time he got a new one."

But I knew that Sam would never make it at the outset of the second visit Parker and I made to Dr. Bushman. (Sam had seen him the day before.) Dr. Hall had evidently been completely right. Stanford, according to Dr. Bushman, wouldn't consider accepting a candidate for a transplant until end-stage heart failure set in. "A transplant is the absolute end resort in the treatment of cardiac disease," he said, "and obviously, because the candidates are so sick when they are accepted into the program, they often die before a heart can be found for them. You must remember always that Sam may well not live to get a heart."

After that it was mostly facts and figures. If Sam did get a heart, his chances of surviving the operation itself were pretty good. His chances of surviving for the first three months after the operation were pretty bad, but "they're improving as every year goes by," Dr. Bushman said.

If Sam could somehow survive that time when rejection and disease were most threatening, the odds slowly began to pick up. If he survived the first six months, his chances of getting through a whole year were better than fifty-fifty.

"When you look at the statistics," Dr. Bushman said, "they seem pretty grim because Stanford has to lump all the early failures in with the successes they're having now. If you just look at the figures from the past four or five years, though, you'll see that the chances for survival are getting greater all the time.

"It's very encouraging on the whole," he finished, and my earlier despair evaporated.

I felt even more encouraged when we got home. Malcolm had sent us a magazine article about the wonderful successes Stanford and Shumway were experiencing, and my confidence soared. I noted, however, at the end of a paragraph, that of the 310 transplants done up to that time throughout the world, only 64 recipients were still alive, and I was miserable all over again.

It was impossible ever to feel encouraged when I looked at Sam. He grew weaker and sicker every day, and every day the paper spit cup he kept next to his bed and next to the sofa in the playroom would be more quickly filled with bloodier and bloodier mucus. Dottie would appear even on her days off to make Jell-O for him, because, as she told me, "You never get it dissolved. You" — with condemnation but total accuracy — "make lumpy Jell-O!"

The ends of the afternoons were always the best. We'd all meet in the kitchen or up in Sam's room if he had a bad day and talk about California. Dottie would tease Sam about "the lengths some people will go to get out of going to school," and Sam would tease Alix, and everybody would tell me I was wrong to hope that Sam could come home for Christmas.

"Hell, Mum," Sam would say, "that's the peak of the accident season. If I came home, I might miss my donor."

Visitors were carefully screened. "God, I hate talking," he'd say, and only when Fred appeared would there be a retreat to the playroom and the sounds of voices over the noise of the stereo and through the closed door. He was always happier after one of Freddie's visits.

On the Saturday night before Thanksgiving, though, two friends from Kent called on the phone at ten o'clock. "He's gone to bed," I said. "Could he call you tomorrow?"

"We're in Cape Elizabeth," they announced. "We're lost."

When they got to the house five minutes later, Parker had gotten Sam up, and the three of us listened to the tale of their pilgrimage. They had left Kent on Friday with the father of one of them and had driven to northern Vermont. That in itself was a five-hour trip. With the father's permission, they had driven five more hours to get to Cape Elizabeth to say good-bye to Sam.

"We gotta leave, though, by six o'clock tomorrow morning," the one who had the car said apologetically. "Dad says we've got to get back to Vermont by eleven so he can drive us back to Kent."

"I guess he does have Kent to back him up," I said to Parker when we finally got to bed that night.

Sam seemed quite well the next day, then had a bad two days on Monday and Tuesday, after which he recuperated enough to announce that of course he was going to Aunt

Roz's for Thanksgiving, and where was the new suit I'd bought him in August?

It was still in the box, and it was the first complete suit he had ever owned. He had instructed me when I went to New York in August that he would like it to be three-piece and pin-striped, and Brooks Brothers had had one, but not in Sam's size. They would order one, they said, alter it to the measurements I had given them, and send it to Sam in September at school.

Sam had left Kent before the suit arrived, and Hart Perry had had it mailed on to us at home, but neither Sam nor I were into suits by the time it reached Cape Elizabeth. On that Wednesday before Thanksgiving, I got it out of the box, Dottie pressed it, and Sam hung it in his closet with all the reverence a matador accords his costume for the ring.

"You won't recognize me when I get all dressed up tomorrow, will you, Mum?" he said when he went to bed, and he was right; I didn't.

Getting dressed for Christmas and Thanksgiving in the Poole household is only achieved by grim determination and concerted poundings on bathroom doors. In the excitement of keeping one pair of stockings for myself and away from Alix and Ruth and of sneaking a white shirt out of Parker's drawer for Malcolm, I had almost forgotten Sam and his new suit. I ran into him in the long narrow hall upstairs, looking at himself in the full-length mirror at one end.

"Christ, Mum," he protested, "what size did you get?"

The thirty-two-inch waist he had had in August must have become twenty-six inches. The pants were hanging halfway down his seat, there was room inside the vest for me as well, and the shoulders of the coat stood a full four inches away from his body on each side.

I couldn't think of anything to say; he looked like a corpse. Rozzie and I had bought a wonderfully handsome necktie for Daddy in New York two days before he died. It was cream-colored and had polo ponies embroidered on it, and it had arrived in Portland the day after he died. Rozzie and I had had him buried in it, and suddenly, looking at Sam, I knew I'd bought more new clothes for a funeral. I could see him all stretched out in a coffin in that horrible blue pin-striped suit.

I gulped and tried to laugh. "Sam, you made the pants too long," I choked out and rushed downstairs.

I don't remember anything about that Thanksgiving dinner at Rozzie and Bill's except for two things. When Uncle Scully, a dear bachelor friend of us all, made his annual toast, "To absent friends," Rozzie and I both had to get up and flee to the kitchen in tears. The other thing I remember was Sam and the scalloped oysters. He had always loved Aunt Roz's oysters more than anything else in the world, and he valiantly ate two helpings, turned pasty white, and asked Charlie to take him home.

I don't even remember washing the dishes with Rozzie, but when I got home Sam was lying in bed with a basin next to his pillow, and Ruthie and Charlie, looking terrified, were sitting nearby.

"How can he stand it?" Ruthie asked me later.

"I don't know" was all I could say; but I did know, though, after the shopping trip I took with Alix the Saturday after Thanksgiving to buy his birthday presents, that his sickness had enveloped every bit and piece of me.

Sam, I had decided, would still be in the hospital when he became eighteen on the third of December, and I wanted to have some presents to take out to California with us. It was hard to know what to buy, but Alix finally found a marvelous collection of T-shirts at a sporting-goods store, and I sorted through the pile until I came upon one with a huge red broken heart on it. I couldn't stop looking at it. The tears started rolling down my cheeks, but I still couldn't put it down.

It's only a joke, I kept saying to myself. Then I heard a voice behind me ask, "How's Sam, Mrs. Poole?" and I turned around to see Dr. Bushman. I dropped the shirt as if I'd been caught reading a dirty book, but all the way home, blushing with shame, I kept wondering if he'd seen what was on the front of it.

Sunday morning was even grimmer. At noon Parker and Uncle Bill went to the old church about a quarter of a mile from the Richardsons' winter house and bought adjoining cemetery plots.

The four of us had always agreed that we wanted to be buried there together. The church overlooked the fields and marshes where Rozzie and I had ridden when we were children and where we skied and walked now with our own, but whenever we had asked Bill and Parker to select our gravesites, they would answer in unison, "We will. We'll give them to you for Christmas."

It stopped being a family joke after we talked to Dr. Bushman. "If he dies, I want him to be somewhere that he knows and loves," I said to Parker. "I want him to be near us here at the Cape."

It took longer than anyone expected, and the rest of us were congregating in the kitchen at our house for the Sunday picnic when Sam dragged downstairs.

"Where are Dad and Uncle Bill?" he asked, and, thank God, Rozzie said, "Oh, I think they had some business thing, didn't they, Aunt Vic?" because I couldn't speak at all.

Pokie drove us to Boston on Monday morning for our flight to California. "That'll make one less plane we'll have to get Sam off and on," Parker said, and he also ordered a wheelchair to meet us at the TWA terminal at Logan Airport in Boston.

It was a grim day to leave home. It was sleeting when we got up and cold and miserable. All the way down to Boston in the car, I kept seeing Rozzie sitting in her nightgown and overcoat in one of the rocking chairs in our kitchen with a crazy old green felt hat of Louise's pulled down over her head. She'd gotten to our house at seven that morning. "Sam can't go all the way out there without a kiss from his aunt," she'd said and had waved us off from the driveway, her nightgown flapping in the wind.

When we got to the terminal, Sam got into the wheelchair without protest. I had expected I-don't-need-its and I-won'ts, but he slumped down into it almost with relief, accepting without comment from Parker the huge manila envelope of X-rays and echograms of the past ten months which Dr. Wakely had directed us to deliver to Stanford. People in wheelchairs always appear to be burdened down with possessions their attendants don't wish to or can't carry, and Sam was no exception. While Parker went off to check the bags through, he sat abjectly — his entire lap hidden under the envelope and his untied Adidas resting awkwardly on the foot supports — sporadically exchanging words with Pokie. I stood beside the two of them, wondering miserably if the three of us would ever be together again.

"See ya, Parker" was all Sam said to Pokie as his father

pushed him off toward our gate, and all Pokie said was, "Yeah, see ya, Sam," as he headed out the door. I turned once to look at him, though. He was still standing in the sleet outside the terminal, watching us through the glass doors.

Chapter Seven

Parker and I had gotten up that morning at four thirty Maine time. Twenty-one hours later we walked into our room at the Holiday Inn in Palo Alto. The fact that it was only ten thirty at night in California did nothing to refresh my spirits, and the Gideon Bible on the bureau didn't either. It was open to a Psalm that said: "I am poured out like water, and all my bones are out of joint."

Oh, King David, me too, I thought, as I closed the Bible and looked up to see myself reflected in the mirror above it. My off-white slacks and sweater that a New York saleslady had assured me would be perfect for California were not only wrinkled, they bore the lurid remains of two cups of coffee and two glasses of red wine. Overcome by enthusiasm to view the Rockies, Parker had twisted in his seat and soaked me from bosom to knee, but my bedraggled and still-damp attire couldn't touch the face above it. Beautiful I am not at the best of times, but the Witch of Endor confronted me that night. My hair hung limp and colorless around a face that it would be a kindness to describe as haggard. My eyes, which are small and deep-set anyway, looked like slits, and the gray circles underneath them sagged and puffed simultaneously. Sackcloth and ashes couldn't have made me a more suitable companion for King David.

Reflected in the mirror behind me, I could see Parker awkwardly sprawled in and over a chair that had never been designed for a six-foot-four-inch frame. If not as soiled as I was, he was at least as rumpled, and his face had its exhausted November-to-April I-need-a-vacation look. His swarthy Latin blood, proudly inherited from some remote French ancestor, does not winter well, and his dashing May-to-October tan had already grayed to a Siberian pallor.

"Look at us," I despaired. "Sam needs knights in shining armor, and all he's got are two worn-out old wrecks. Oh, Pa, I'm so scared."

He hoisted most of himself back into the confines of the chair and pulled a cigarette out of the breast pocket of his shirt. "It's been one hell of a day," he said, fumbling in his jacket for a match, "but at least we're here. I know it's scary as hell, but if anything can be done for Sam, it's at that hospital. At least it's better than being at home doing nothing. And Sammy's tough, Vic. He'll pass those tests and he'll get a heart. I'd put money on it."

I wanted so much to believe him, but I kept hearing the words of the young intern at Stanford who had taken Sam's case history that afternoon: "We can't afford to give a heart to someone who hasn't got a good chance of surviving. Hearts are scarce. We can't waste them." The thought that Sam might already be too sick to get a heart had never crossed my mind until that afternoon, and now it obliterated everything else.

We had been in grand spirits when we got to Stanford. Our flight to San Francisco had been uneventful, other than the coffee-and-wine debacle, and no one had been more surprised than Parker at my sanguine approach to the accident.

"It's not like you not to be mad," he had said, and it wasn't, but somehow I hadn't felt a bit like me either in all that off-white smartness. It had been a relief to be considerably less than perfect again.

The unaccustomed splendors of first class and the attentions paid us, thanks to our patient and his huge manila envelope of X-rays and records, made all three of us feel important and purposeful. A wheelchair met us at the plane, and, in a flood of California sunshine and a rented car of an exotic yellow rarely seen in Maine, we started south down the freeway to Palo Alto.

On November 7 we had been sent a letter from a Miss H. Knott of the Cardiology Division at Stanford. She had enclosed maps, indicating with red arrows the best route for us to follow, and Sam, sitting in the front seat with Parker, appointed himself their sole interpreter.

In her letter, Miss Knott confirmed that a bed had been booked for Sam on the cardiology service for November 29 and suggested that we admit him through the emergency entrance so that he would not have to wait at the regular admitting office. For this bit of consideration for Sam, I had loved the unseen Miss Knott on the spot. Though I was uncomfortably wedged in the back seat beside and beneath our belongings, my admiration for her knew no bounds as we got off at the proper Palo Alto exit and found ourselves surrounded by signs directing us to Stanford University Medical Center.

"Hey, you guys," I kept mumbling up from under the luggage, "look at the flowers. Look, they're planting pansies and it's November! It doesn't look like almost Christmastime at all."

Sam had taken a more sophisticated approach to the landscape and made little comment, but just as I spotted a sign on the left saying STANFORD UNIVERSITY MEDICAL CENTER — EMERGENCY, he spotted another on the right saying *Saks Fifth Avenue.*

"Look, Mum," he said, "There's Saks. You can get your Erno out here!"

"How can we lose?" Parker declared as he turned left and left again, following the red arrows to Emergency. "Sam's going to get a heart; you've got your Erno. I guess we'll have to close down our Maine operations permanently."

Abandoning our car in a covered concrete tunnel that strongly reminded me of a gun emplacement, we came, molelike, up some steps to find ourselves in a very small and very unintimidating waiting room.

Within seconds Sam was trundled off in a wheelchair, with Parker and me following behind, and swiftly bedded down in a room on West I-B, the cardiology service. It was a tiny semiprivate room directly opposite the nurses' station, and Sam's section of it was entirely chairless. For a minute or two, I busied myself putting away the T-shirts and underdrawers that Sam insisted were the only proper attire for hospitalization, Parker leaned against the wall in a futile attempt to take up less space, and the patient himself started muttering about ice.

"Absolutely no," said a nurse. "Ice is very bad for cardiac patients. No violent temperature changes," but then, noticing the anguished look on Sam's face, she added, "I'll check with one of the doctors for you later."

After that we were too busy to even think about ice or the lack of it. Sam had been stowed into bed at about four o'clock, and by five we had been visited by multitudinous nurses, interns, and residents; by Dr. John Schroeder, the chief cardiologist for the Stanford Transplant Program, who had set up everything for us through Dr. Wakely; and by Miss H. Knott herself.

They all introduced themselves so cheerfully — "Hello, I'm so-and-so, I'm a member of the cardiology team here at Stanford" — that even I, who have made a lifetime occupation of icily avoiding connections with teams of any sort, could not but thaw. There seemed, however, to be an alarming lack of surnames, and I was at a loss to know how you communicated with people. It didn't seem quite proper to pursue a nurse down the corridor yelling "Hey, Susie," so the arrival of Miss Knott, who could easily have been taken for a Bostonian and might even have been somewhere around my age, was a great relief.

"Miss Knott, what should we do about finding an apartment here in Palo Alto?" I asked, and her answer produced the first hint that our day was about to crumble to pieces.

"Oh, my," Miss Knott said gently, "I shouldn't do anything at all until you find out whether Sam will be accepted as a transplant recipient. If he is, I'll be delighted to help you."

I remember wondering briefly what she meant by "if" Sam was accepted, but instantly decided that she must mean whether he was sick enough to be and put the matter out of my mind.

I don't think Dr. Schroeder said "if" at all. He told us that someone would detail the tests Sam would undergo to determine his condition, that another catheterization would be done, probably on Wednesday, and that of course every possible method of correcting his disease with drugs or surgically without transplantation would be explored. He asked us a few questions about the history of Sam's heart condition, said we would see him later, and departed.

Just as the clatterings and bangings of dinner trays started outside in the hall, a young woman who introduced herself as "Pat, I'm an intern on the cardiology team here at Stanford," appeared at the foot of Sam's bed. Armed with pads, papers, lists, and charts, she immediately endeared herself to us by procuring two chairs and proved her obvious scientific merit by finding places in that minuscule room to put them. She sat down and started off a barrage of questions about family diseases, beginning with Sam's and progressing backward unto those of the third and fourth generations.

Parker not only has no idea what any of his relatives died of, he is even shaky on grandparental names. Petty enough to feel smug, I accounted for them all, and in general the lungs, livers, kidneys, and hearts seemed to pass muster. The senility that runs rampant through both sides of the family apparently didn't distress her a bit, although she did express concern that Daddy had died of an arterial hemorrhage in his leg. When I assured her, however, that he'd caused it himself by doctoring the leg with antiquated carbolated Vaseline, according to a prescription from his medical bible, *Diseases of Man and Beast*, she laughed and went on with her questions.

"What about herpes?" she asked.

I was very familiar with that particular virus because Mother had had shingles and always suffered from cold sores. It seemed that it was not in Sam's favor that she had.

Herpes is one of the plagues of the heart transplant recipient, and it was definitely a blessing that her susceptibility had not been passed on to me or the children.

Pat put down her pencil. "You see, " she said, "if Sam were historically prone to herpes, or diabetes, or any other complicating disease, it would be foolish for us to even contemplate a transplant for him."

It would be equally futile, she explained, to contemplate one if his lungs, liver, or kidneys were already irreversibly damaged, and the tests he would have during the week would establish the condition of those organs. Psychiatric tests would determine if he had the necessary strength and will to endure and if Parker and I would be able to give him the support he would so desperately need.

"If Sam is accepted at the end of this evaluation," she said, "it will mean that he will go into surgery with decent odds. It's the only way we can make this program work." That was when she said, absolutely matter-of-factly, "We can't afford to give a heart to someone who hasn't got a good chance of surviving. Hearts are scarce. We can't waste them."

Terror seized me. I was standing, leaning against the wall at the foot of Sam's bed, and to keep from showing my distress I looked down toward the floor. The stains on my slacks and sweater, which had seemed quite subtle in the bright California sunshine, looked garish and disgusting, but, raising my head to avoid them, I was confronted by Sam's feet. They were protruding, bony and bluish gray, from either side of the sheet.

Princess Volupine extends a meagre, blue-nailed, phthisic hand. The words came into my mind again as clearly as though I had the poem in front of me. Phthisic, I thought to myself. He's phthisic just like that girl in Dr. Owens's office. Sam looks just the way she did. Oh, dear God, what if it's too late?

The rest of our interview with Pat became a blur. I had seen a copy of the letter Dr. Wakely had written to Stanford in which he stated that Sam would "ultimately be in need of cardiac transplantation," and to me "ultimately" had meant "later on." I was fully prepared to wait anywhere or for any length of time until that moment came, but, although I knew he might die waiting for the right heart to come along, I had never dreamt he could be too sick to even qualify to wait. I knew that Lois Christopherson, the heart transplant social-service worker, had said over the phone to Parker, "If Sam were judged to be a suitable candidate," but the "if" had been an uncrossed bridge in my mind, as I found it had been in Parker's.

I saw Pat stand up to go, and I remember hearing her say, "At the end of this week, we'll know exactly how things stand. You'd better be prepared for a battery of tests, though, Sam. They want to really check you out. I'll see you later." She started out the door and then turned back with a smile. "Oh, yes, they say you want ice. Yes, Sam, you can have all the ice you want. It's only people with heart attacks who can't. I'll tell the nurses' station."

We watched Sam not eat his dinner and watched him watch television; we chatted with his roommate and speculated with Sam himself about the psychiatric tests we'd have.

"Think up some really weird ones for the inkblots, Sam; they might decide you're a genius," I said as we went out, but in the car I clutched Parker.

"What if it's too late?" I said. "Oh, God, Parker, what will we do?" and I kept it up until we finally checked in at the Holiday Inn.

I spent a good part of the night, after Parker finally fell asleep, in the bathroom, trying to read. I couldn't connect one sentence to another; all I could think about was Sam and the letter Bill Scott had written from Vanderbilt to Dr. Shumway on October 25.

Parker had written Bill Scott when we took Sam home from the hospital on October 8, asking him to write Dr. Shumway about Sam. Dr. Wakely had written Dr. Shumway on October 12. Nothing more had happened until October 28, when Parker got a letter back from Bill Scott saying that he had been away at a medical meeting and had just gotten home. He enclosed a copy of a letter he had written to Dr. Shumway on the same day. Presumably Dr. Shumway had received his letter toward the end of the week as we had, because on Monday morning Dr. Schroeder had called Dr. Wakely from Stanford and suggested that Sam come out to California.

How long Dr. Wakely's letter would have gone unanswered without Bill Scott's "Dear Norm" appeal to Dr. Shumway had occasioned great speculation and hilarity at our November picnics. "You know what happened," Rozzie would exclaim. "Dr. Shumway got Bill Scott's letter and paged Dr. Schroeder on the spot. 'I sent a letter down to your office last week, John, from a Dr. Philip Wakely in Portland, Maine, about a kid named Talcott Poole. He's the nephew of a colleague of mine. Get in touch with him. We need that boy!'"

Sitting in the bathroom that night, I didn't find it funny at all. Bill Scott is actually my cousin-in-law; it is Mary, his wife, who is my blood relation. Absurd as it sounds now, I kept thinking to myself all that night, Oh, God, what if Mary hadn't married Bill Scott? What if Bill hadn't come home from his trip? Dear God, what would have happened if we didn't know anybody?

Finally one last question, more terrifying than any of the others, came into my head. I couldn't stand to ask it to myself, and at four I went back into the bedroom to wake up Parker, who was already awake.

"Parker," I said, "what if we'd believed Dr. Hall?"

When Pokie fell in the cesspool years ago, I speedily discovered that nothing dispels the terrors of the night like hospital routine. It is almost impossible to believe that death would dare intrude upon the awesome regularity of the meals, the baths, the tests, and the medicine schedule. It was very comforting to sit in Sam's room in the midst of routine and it was even more comforting to meet Lois Christopherson.

She came to Sam's room at about eleven on Tuesday morning in a white coat, pleated wool skirt, and marvelously unsensible shoes. "Hi," she said, "I'm Lois. Are you the Pooles?"

Although it rapidly became evident that Lois in fact was eminently sensible, her hair bounced and her eyes twinkled and she was not in the least formidable. For the better part of the morning, Sam had been repeatedly wheeled in and out of the room for tests. In between, his father had been teaching him to play cribbage, and Sam had finally collapsed, exhausted, on his pillow. He took one head-twisted glance at Lois, though, sat up eagerly, and stuck out his hand. "Hi," he said. "I'm Sam."

Before we could even offer one of our treasured chairs, she had whisked one away from Sam's roommate's side of the room and sat down with jauntily crossed legs and a smile that made me feel as if we'd brought Sam to California to have his tonsils out.

"I've been dying to meet you, Sam," she said, "ever since I talked to your father that first night on the telephone and he told me you were right there in the room with him. I couldn't believe it. I knew right then that you were the kind of person we wanted as a heart transplant candidate."

Lois spoke so positively I felt as though Sam were already a recipient-in-waiting, and my terrible night seemed absurd as long as she was in the room. If I had lost everyone I loved, my last penny to boot, and were rapidly and simultaneously going deaf, dumb, and blind in a state institution, I would somehow marshal my waning faculties and summon Lois Christopherson. Somewhere along the line, she had met and conquered despair, and, although in her absence it still dogged the footsteps of her transplant flock, a talk with her could vanquish it again. She never for a minute suggested, however, that it was not an ever-present enemy constantly to be battled.

"You know already, Sam," she said, "that if you had a long life ahead of you, or if we could find some way to control your disease with medicine, we wouldn't want you to be a part of our program. We're delighted with the results we're having with our recipients, but you always have to remember that a heart transplant is a last-ditch stand. I'll bet, though," she added with a smile, "that even a last-ditch stand would look pretty good to you by now, if it could make you feel any better. Right now I guess you feel cold all the time, and it must hurt to do everything. It probably even hurts you to breathe, doesn't it?"

"Oh, God, yes," Sam said. "If I could just take a deep breath again or just walk without it hurting, I'd be happy."

Lois promptly told him he'd be silly to settle for that,

and her words pushed the specter of a Sam too sick to qualify for the transplant program even farther into the shadows. "You'll be able to do almost everything you've ever done before once you get a new heart," she said. "The minute your old one comes out, you'll be warm all over again. A heart transplant is honestly like watching Lazarus rise up from the dead; it's a miracle."

All three of us were staring at her spellbound as she talked.

"If things go well," she went on, "you'll be lifting weights before you're even out of intensive care, and by next summer you could be swimming and playing tennis again just as if you'd never been sick."

I was so excited I couldn't contain myself. "Oh, Sam," I interrupted, "it sounds just like Cinderella going to the ball. Your pumpkin's going to turn into a coach and your Adidas will turn into glass slippers!"

Sam ignored me, but Lois laughed. "That's right," she said, "but conversely, though, everything can switch back again just as easily. A heart transplant is something you have to fight to get, and you have to fight for the rest of your life to keep it. Let me explain the whole process to you so you'll really understand."

No one, she said, was accepted as a heart transplant recipient who had more than a few months left to live. If Sam were accepted into the Stanford program, he would start that very minute with the first stage of getting a heart, waiting for one. In many ways, Lois said, it was the hardest time of all. It could last for days, weeks, or months. "Or," she added, "as you've been told, it can happen that a heart won't be found for you in time.

"The worse thing of all," she went on, "is not knowing when your heart will come. Every time your telephone rings you're going to expect it to be your heart, but so many times it won't be, you'll probably be totally unprepared when it finally does appear." One candidate, she told us, patiently bathed and shaved every day for three months so that he would always be in a presentable state to arrive at the hospital. Thoroughly disgusted, he woke up one morning and decided to abandon his ablutions. It was, of course, the day his heart came. "You can't win," Lois said, "but that's Stage One."

Stage Two, it seemed, was actually the easy part. The operation of transferring one person's heart to another is far simpler and less hazardous than a coronary artery bypass, for example, and most people live through it to wake up warm and, best of all, feeling alive for probably the first time in years.

The words Sam had said to me that awful August morning at the cottage came rushing back. "Oh, Mum. . . . I wish I could get up in the morning and just say, 'I feel good.' You know, like it's going to be a nice day." Without any warning, my eyes filled with tears at the incredible possibility of me saying "How do you feel, darling?" and Sam saying "Great!" and I sniffed, I'm ashamed to say, audibly.

Lois didn't seem to mind. "It's absolutely ridiculous," she said, laughing. "Here are these heart transplants who've had their chests cut wide open and their rib cages forced apart, and they all wake up and say they feel fine — no chest pain at all.

"It's a measure of what they've endured before surgery," she said more soberly, "and it's frightening to us to think of just what they have endured. Even if a recipient should die after that first day, he will often say before he does that that first moment of feeling alive again was worth everything."

Ignoring the fact that his bed wasn't even cranked up to support his back, Sam leaned forward eagerly. "Oh, God," he said, "that would be so great. I don't care about the pain. Pain you can live with; you get over it. It's just being sick and not doing anything about it that doesn't make sense."

Lois smiled at him. "I know, Sam," she said. "that's what all our transplants say, but I'm glad you understand about pain because in Stage Three you'll be faced with a lot more of it. That's the time you'll be in the intensive care unit, or ICU, as we call it, and it really bugs some of our transplants. To begin with, for one month or more you'll be completely isolated from the outside world, but at the same time you won't even have the consolation of privacy. A nurse will be in your room monitoring everything you do, twenty-four hours a day, regardless of whether or not your father or mother is there. Everyone who comes into your room will be masked, gowned, hatted, booted, and gloved, and you won't be able to tell one person from another. You can't imagine how horrid it is to want to have someone you love touch you and then realize that the only way they can is through those clammy plastic gloves. It can drive you bananas."

Nothing she could say could dampen Sam. "I don't care how clammy anybody feels as long as I feel warm," he said. "Is that all I have to worry about?"

It wasn't; medicines and shots were still unaccounted for. Prednisone, the staple drug for all transplants, had miserable side effects, Lois said. Not only did it tend to make you chipmunk-cheeked and potbellied, it made you wildly hungry all the time, and any weight gain in transplants had to be carefully monitored. It also caused wild mood swings from elation to depression and back again which were disconcerting and troublesome. Imuran, another drug, caused bone marrow depression and a decrease in white blood cells.

It seemed that, as Dr. Wakely had told us, there would be a mélange of drugs that Sam would be taking from the moment he landed in ICU, and he would have to take many of them forever. While none were without their peculiarities and hazards, there was no question that the most helpful medication to the new heart-transplant recipient, but also the most painful of all, was ATG — anti-thymocyte globulin. It would be injected each night "and it's thick, and you have to have huge amounts of it, and it hurts!" Lois said emphatically. "You can't imagine how it hurts. The ATG is injected directly into the thigh, and it actually causes the muscle to break down."

Sam just shrugged and stuck out a thin but still sturdy leg from under the sheets. "Look," he said proudly. "It'll take a lot of that junk to break that muscle down, and I haven't done any exercise at all for months."

"You're right," Lois said with appropriate admiration. "That's great. And it's not as bleak as it sounds. The whole process is reversible. You'll start therapy just as soon as possible to build what muscle you lose back up again. You're lucky to start with all that muscle, though, Sam. Some of our transplants have such skinny legs when they start that the nurses say they almost cry at the thought of having to inject the ATG into them. Oh, and speaking of nurses, Sam," she said, "you've already got one signed up for you."

Sam smiled. "I guess it doesn't make much difference if she's good-looking or not, if she has to wear all that stuff in my room. Is she nice?"

Lois nodded. "And good-looking too," she said. "You'll meet her before the operation, so you can judge for yourself."

She told us that the disorientation transplant recipients experienced in ICU from their masked-and-gowned visitors and their isolation had been a terrible problem. Every eight hours when a new shift of nurses came on, a new and unrecognizable form would enter the transplant's room. The transplant team had recently decided that each recipient would have one nurse who signed on for him or her for the duration of the time in ICU. The transplant would have at least one known voice, one person who knew him and his likes and dislikes, one person with whom to share the day's problems.

Sam's nurse was to be Lynn Honma. "She's a darling," Lois said. "She's young and she's pretty, and she signed up for you the minute I told her about you. Somehow I didn't think you'd go for a motherly type, and Lynn's only twenty-four. She's from Hawaii. If you're accepted into the program, she'll come to visit you, as I said, before you get your heart, and if there's anything you can't stand or that really gripes you, tell her then. You won't be able to the day of your operation.

"Lynn can help you a lot," she went on, "because those months in ICU are never easy. That's when you'll probably have your first rejection, and it will probably be a bad one. For some crazy reason, the younger you are — and you, Sam, could be the second-youngest transplant we've ever done — the stronger the rejection seems to be. You may even completely reject your first heart and have to wait for a second one. It happens once in a while, but don't worry. We can keep the bad one going quite a while, and once you've become a recipient, you're automatically Number One on the waiting list. Somehow we always manage to find that second heart if we need it."

I was strangely reminded of the prince in the fairy tale who had seven perils to triumph over before he could claim the princess who lived at the top of the mountain of glass. Lois continued to talk about stages, but they became Sam's princely perils to me. It was all "if": if Sam got accepted, if he survived his wait, if he survived his operation to wake up with a new heart, if he survived his rejections — and then suddenly Lois was producing yet another "if."

"The reason for all the gowning and masking in ICU, Sam," she explained, "is to cut down on the infection factor. You'll be so susceptible to anything that comes along during that time, because of the immunosuppressant drugs you'll be taking, that a sniffle, for example, could turn into pneumonia."

If, after everything else, Sam survived the disease factor, he would go to a recuperative section of the hospital where he would learn to take care of himself and would at long last have the dignity of a little privacy. That stage too could be fraught with rejection and infection, Lois said, and discouragement, and it accounted for the fifth peril. The sixth one was if, at the end of a month or two, Sam were progressing well, he could move to an apartment near the hospital to try living in the unantiseptic world again.

The seventh peril, the final "if," was getting home. Home for me was too far away at the top of the glass mountain to even contemplate, but Lois must have seen it scaled many times. "When you're back home again, Sam," she said, as if it were the logical conclusion for all transplants and princes, "you'll be able to do almost everything you want to do, as I told you, but you'll do it under the rules you've learned from us. Number One: you will have to exercise every day."

We all burst out laughing. "But that's all I want to do," Sam said. "I only wish I could."

"You will," said Lois with assurance, "but you're talking about now. You may get bored with the idea after you get your heart, and you can't. Number Two," she continued, "is that you will have to be careful about going out in public without wearing a mask over your nose and mouth to prevent your picking up germs, and you'll wear one at home if anyone in the house has a cold."

I nervously twisted in my seat to see how that sat with Sam, but he registered no surprise or dismay at all. He just sat there hanging on every word Lois said.

The third rule was that he would probably never again be able to swim in the ocean. There was too much pollution, Lois said; chlorinated pools only were allowable. Still there was no protest from Sam.

"And Number Four," Lois continued, "is that contact sports will be absolutely out for you for good. You'll be taking blood thinners that will make you virtually a hemophiliac, and one good bump could start a hemorrhage."

Sam only laughed. "That's okay," he said. "I never liked playing football all that much anyway; it's an awful lot of work. I can take all those rules. What else?"

It was the final rule that wounded him, the diet he would have to follow for the rest of his life: no salt, no sugar, no cholesterol. "No more pizzas?" he asked wistfully.

"One every six months," Lois directed. "And that's the end of the rules. The only other thing you should know about are the donors. You'll never know whose heart you get, Sam. It's bound to be someone young, because we almost never accept hearts from anyone over thirty, and we'll tell you the donor's sex and exact age, but we can't tell you any more. We've found that there are too many emotional complications on both sides if the donor's family or the recipient know any more than that."

She paused a minute. "You know," she said, "I have such a deep respect for the donor families. Someone they love — probably their child — has died in what is usually a terrible accident, and all you would normally expect them to think about is their grief. Instead, they somehow manage to think of someone with a problem like yours. It's awesome, the courage of these people. You can thank the family of whoever it is who ultimately gives you your heart through me, and they will know from me how wonderful is the gift they have given you. It *is* a gift, though, Sam, with no strings attached. The heart is yours."

There was nothing any of us could say. We all sat there quietly for a minute or two, and then Lois looked at her watch and jumped up. "Good Lord," she said, "I'm half an hour late for a meeting," and her solemnity vanished. "It's been great meeting you all. See you later, Sam."

"Apartments?" I asked. "Should we start looking for one?"

"Oh, I forgot," she said. "Here you are," and she handed me a thick booklet. "That's filled with all the hotels, motels, and apartment houses around here. If Sam's accepted, you ought to start looking around. Good-bye."

After she left, Sam's energy subsided and he collapsed to his usual position: flat on his back. The afternoon, interspersed by tests, passed without event. He had lung scans and liver scans; he had blood tests and X-rays. Members of the transplant team appeared singly and in droves to poke and prod and query, and they all appeared to me to be alarmingly young and even more alarmingly bearded. When the cardiologist who was to do Sam's catheterization left the room, I could not suppress an "Oh, my God, he looks just like one of Pokie's friends," and it was not entirely meant as a compliment.

We were told that we wouldn't be able to see Sam on Wednesday until late in the morning. He would be moved to an intensive care room down the hall after the catheterization so that his heart could be monitored for a day or so. They were going to experiment with different drugs, which would be given intravenously to see if his heart condition could be in any way corrected without, as Dr. Shumway would say, "the ultimate therapeutic intervention of heart transplantation."

Parker determined that we would use the morning to apartment hunt, and, prodded by him, I made arrangements over the telephone Tuesday night for us to look at three.

"What if Sam isn't accepted?" I said to Parker the next morning, looking up from a map I was trying to decipher, as we drove off to our first apartment.

"He will be," Parker said. "And why do you always say 'Turn right' when you mean 'Turn left'? It's very confusing."

By eleven thirty, despite my directional flaws, we returned to the hospital, having seen three apartments inside and out. When we found Sam in his intensive care room, we forgot about them all. The room was identical to the one he had departed, except that it was equipped with such a variety of esoteric machinery that there was even less floor space. The bed near the window was empty; on the one near the door I could distinguish a male patient, but he didn't look at all like Sam to me. He looked like a sick old man.

"That's not Sam," I muttered to Parker. "We've got the wrong room."

Two doctors and a nurse were bent over the bed. Evidently hearing my voice, one of the doctors looked up and said, "Are you Sam's parents? His bladder closed up after the heart catheterization for some reason, and we're having a little trouble getting a urinary catheter inserted. Could you wait outside for a little while?"

I took one last agonized look at the patient I hadn't recognized. He didn't make a sound, but it was evident from the way he was twisting and squirming on the bed amid a tangle of wires and IV tubes that he was in considerable discomfort. It still didn't look like Sam to me, but I retreated to the lounge at the end of the hall to wait with Parker.

"There's not an inch of that poor boy that's going to be left unviolated," I protested vehemently. "No one who's only seventeen should have to endure all this." But that was the only motherly protest I ever made in defense of Sam's personal dignity the entire time he was at Stanford.

By three in the afternoon, Sam's bladder was itself again. He had stopped looking like an unfamiliar old man to me, and we'd adjusted to all his tubes and wires. Above and behind his head was his cardiac monitoring machine, which he couldn't turn to see but which was great fun to watch and describe to him. With every beat of his heart, there would be a beep and little lights would trace a bewilderingly erratic course across a screen.

"It's just like playing TV tennis," I was exclaiming with fascination, when a new patient was wheeled into the room on a stretcher and deposited on the empty bed near the window. It was only after the stretcher bearers had departed that I realized that the patient was a she.

I nudged Parker, and he nudged Sam, and all three of us looked at each other and simply shrugged. Stanford sophistication was already making a dent on our New England proprieties.

She was quite obviously very sick, and in the two-and-a-half days that she was Sam's roommate I never heard her speak at all. She appeared to be middle-aged and very frail, but she was lovely looking. By Thursday I had decided that her bare backside, often inadvertently exposed as she turned on her bed, would not corrupt Sam's morals. By Friday I had added her to my list of nightly sitting-in-the-bathroom worries, hoping for Sam's sake that she would not die when he was alone with her in the room, and for hers that Stanford would quickly find out what was wrong with her heart and correct it.

Friday itself was Sam's birthday. Sometime during the afternoon, his tubes and wires were removed and a telegram arrived from Aunt Roz and Uncle Bill saying DON'T BE HEARTLESS. WE'RE PUMPING FOR YOU, but on the whole it was hardly a celebrational day. The two T-shirts, the book, the bathrobe, and the Timex watch we gave him seemed hardly celebrational either, but even though the day was as woe-filled as any poor Wednesday's child could possibly expect, Sam never complained. He kissed me and shook Parker's hand, and announced that it was a great satisfaction to think that he could now drink legally.

"That's not all, Sam," Parker said. "If you get accepted for a heart, you can sign all the hospital forms yourself," but that thought unfortunately brought up a new anxiety.

When Sam had been admitted, we had gathered that his

tests would be completed by the end of the week. Here it was, though, late Friday afternoon, and we had no idea at all how far he had progressed in the evaluation process.

Were the medical tests finished? We didn't know. Had he done well or badly? Again, the same answer. What we did know, though, was that the psychological exams still lay ahead of us. Not one of us could recollect a question being asked or a word spoken that smacked of anything psychiatric. It was very depressing having no idea when or if Sam would be able to leave the hospital, and the sound of the woman in the next bed gently gasping for breath through an oxygen mask could hardly be construed as encouraging.

I was just saying, with a confidence I didn't feel, "Oh, well, they'll probably do them on Monday, and then we'll know one way or the other," when Dr. Schroeder entered the room, followed by a retinue of white coats. Parker and I immediately abandoned our chairs and pushed back against the sink and the closet to accommodate the multitudes clustered around Sam's bed. I remember recognizing Pat, the intern who took Sam's case history, and the bearded cardiologist who looked like a friend of Pokie's, but otherwise memory fades in a blur of clinical coats and bristling mustaches.

Everyone looked very solemn, and I suddenly knew that they had come to tell us Sam was too sick to get a heart. They'd decided not to bother with the psychological tests because, medically, he was just too sick. I felt my throat get all tight, but I just stood there clenching my teeth.

"Sam," Dr. Schroeder said, "there's absolutely no way we can correct your heart condition with any drugs or any form of surgery. We've tried everything we can, and there's just no way it will improve anything at all."

I clutched the sink behind me with icy-cold hands and stood there with my clenched teeth, staring at him.

"We've been very concerned," he went on, "because we discovered almost immediately that you have suffered some lung and liver damage already, but it appears," he said, with the first glimmer of a smile, "to be entirely reversible with drugs. We've just had a meeting of the cardiac transplant team, and we've decided that you would make an excellent transplant recipient. You've been accepted into the program."

Thank God there were so many people around Sam's bed or I should have made a complete fool of myself. I always do when something wonderful has happened. I wanted to hug Dr. Schroeder, I wanted to throw my arms around Sam and cry "Oh, it *is* your birthday," but, mercifully for my dignity, I couldn't move. I felt tears running down my cheeks, and I settled for grabbing Parker's hand and squeezing it as hard as I could.

I remember Sam shaking Dr. Schroeder's hand and Dr. Schroeder saying that Sam could leave the hospital the next day to wait for a heart in the area, and that he wanted to talk to Parker and me that night after rounds or the next morning before Sam was discharged. And finally I remember Sam asking Pat, our intern, who was last in line to leave the room, "But what about the psychological tests? Will I have to come back into the hospital to have them?"

"You had them," Pat said. "You passed. Isn't that great?" and she left the room smiling, without a word of explanation.

Oddly enough, it was what happened to the woman in the next bed that explained Stanford's psychiatric-testing system to us. At about nine that night, Parker was out of the room, pacing the halls in a fruitless search for Dr. Schroeder, Sam was almost asleep, and only the light in the entranceway of the room was on. In the semidarkness a bell began to ring somewhere behind the far bed.

Oh, God, I thought, something's gone wrong with her machines. She was still be-tubed and be-wired, and I fled to the door of the room crying, "Help! That lady's bells are ringing."

A doctor rushed by me into the room, picked up an innocently baby-blue telephone from the floor behind her bed, and, with a withering glance at me, answered it. "It's for you, Sam," he said and, handing him the receiver, departed with disdain.

It appeared, from the sounds the receiver was emitting, to be the entire sixth form of Kent School calling to wish Sam a happy birthday, and Sam had to lean practically into the adjacent bed to reach the phone at all. "Hey, you guys, what's up?" he roared while the woman quivered visibly.

"Shhh," I kept saying to no avail. He had to tell each and every friend that he'd been accepted. "I'm all psyched up," he kept saying. "I can't wait. I just wanna get going."

I had to put the receiver back on the telephone for him, and as I did I caught a glimpse of her face. Her body had evidently reacted only by instinct to all Sam's noise. Her face registered nothing but a remote and profound sadness that seemed to have no association with us at all.

The next morning another, but smaller, group of white coats entered the room, this time bypassing Sam's bed.

"Mrs. Turner," said one of the doctors gently, and then again, "Mrs. Turner?" — a little louder, as if to attract her attention. She gave no indication that she was listening to him, but he said, "I'm sorry, but after consultation we don't feel that a cardiac transplantation for you can be justified. Is there any way we can help to make arrangements for your care when you get back to Los Angeles?"

I was staring openly. I had gotten so involved that I wanted her to protest or to cry out, but the only sign she gave that she had comprehended what he said was a slow denying shake of her head, and the doctors departed. I remember thinking with horror, How could they? How could they just sentence her to death like that? And it wasn't until much later that I finally understood that what they had done was a kindness.

The entire episode could have been lifted out of a Kafka novel. It ruined the day. Sam had witnessed the whole thing, and, although he said nothing then, afterward he lay silent and withdrawn, abandoning even the Saturday morning TV cartoons. Parker still couldn't find Dr. Schroeder, and finally he directed me to wait in the lounge at the end of the hall to see if I could spot our mentor coming or going. I couldn't, and instead I found myself sitting next to the woman's brother. We had talked back and forth while she shared Sam's room, and he had been sitting with her when Sam was accepted. He had been sitting with her too when she was told she couldn't qualify for a heart.

"I'm sorry," I said stupidly.

"No," he said, "it's a blessing. She's a nurse; she knows the score. And it isn't just that she has a bad heart. She has nothing to live for. Her husband is dead and her two sons aren't any good. One of them is too busy to see her, and the other one's stolen everything she owned. It would be cruel to put her through the whole business of a heart transplant; she'd never make it. All she has is me and her two sisters, and we're nowhere near her. We live up near the mother lode."

I still wonder almost daily about the woman and her two dreadful sons, although I'm sure she's long since dead, and I still wonder fruitlessly why I never asked where the mother lode was; but after that morning I never wondered again about the psychological tests. I could hear Sam telling his friends at Kent, "I'm all psyched up," and I knew the message had gotten through to the cardiac transplant team.

We didn't take Sam home from the hospital that day after all. No one seemed to know where Dr. Schroeder was, and I could tell that Parker was getting upset. Good ex-Marine that he is, Parker is a great believer in marching orders. He gives them to me and the children; he expects to be given them by doctors. No one had told anyone which medicines Sam was to continue with or which he was to stop taking, and here we were supposed to take him home — if a Holiday Inn can be called home — before lunch.

Parker was beginning to mutter ("This is a hell of a way to run a railroad") in the hall outside Sam's door, and I was beginning to detach myself from the entire problem by watching passersby, when a rather rumpled young man with no white coat appeared beside us.

"I'm Dr. Clusen," he said cheerfully. "You can take Sam home any time now."

Dr. Clusen couldn't have been a day older than Malcolm, and unfortunately for him, poor dear, he bore a startling resemblance to a friend of Malcolm's who had been trying to find himself since the troubles of the sixties began. Parker glowered at him as if he were actually Malcolm's friend. "I thought we were going to see Dr. Schroeder either last night or this morning," he growled. "What about Sam's medicines? Nobody's given us any directions at all."

Dr. Clusen opened his mouth in preparation for speech, but he wasn't quick enough. Parker wouldn't wait.

"I'm not taking Sam anywhere," he said, "until somebody tells us exactly what to do."

"He's trying to, Parker," I said.

Suddenly I became aware of a noise from Sam's room. I stuck my head in the door and saw that he was sitting up in bed with his mouth open as if he were trying to call. His lips wouldn't move, and the only sound that came out was "—ad."

I turned back to the hall. "Parker," I said, "stop it. Sam's not going anywhere; he's got a migraine. He's trying to call you."

Any resemblance between Malcolm's friend who couldn't find himself and Dr. Clusen vanished on the spot. In seconds he had checked Sam, produced the medicines he needed for his headache, cranked down his bed, and become Parker's hero.

Dr. Clusen agreed with me that Sam wasn't going anywhere until his migraine subsided, and Parker and I retreated on foot — to the outdoor café near the hospital that had become our lunch headquarters — to regroup. It was a cloudy, dispirited day, which matched our mood exactly, but we did manage to settle on an apartment before we'd finished our coffee.

We'd seen four more possibilities since our initial foray on the day of Sam's catheterization. Memories of the storehouse at home, bulging with the contents of Mother and Daddy's kitchens and linen closets, had made my New England conscience agree with Parker's that it would be wicked to buy one thing in California and that fully furnished was the only way to go. That cut the seven we had looked at down to four. I refused to live in one of them on the grounds that it reminded me of the Garden of Allah, where poor Scott Fitzgerald spend his last alcoholic days, and another would have bankrupted us in short order. That left only two we could possibly consider.

"I think we should take the first one we looked at," Parker said, swallowing the last of his coffee. "I like the exposure." Remembering that this was exactly what he had said when he selected Camp Bruin, I knew the die was cast, for better or for worse.

We committed ourselves to Mrs. McNutt, our new landlady, that afternoon over the telephone. She said we could rent the apartment on a monthly basis, could move in as soon as the curtains were cleaned — mandated by California law, it seemed — and feeling secure, if not elated, we went back to the hospital.

There was a message waiting for us from Dr. Schroeder, explaining that he had been tied up in an emergency and giving us his home phone number. Parker got hold of him that night, and at ten the next morning we met him in the lounge at the end of Sam's hall.

I'm a big believer in pathetic fallacy; whatever the weather is doing, I'm doing too. As we walked up to the hospital that morning, the sun was shining, primroses and pansies were blooming everywhere, and the fountains in front of the hospital were spurting jets of diamonds up into the air. Dr. Schroeder smiled at us so warmly and was so enthusiastic about Sam that even though disease, danger, and death were the chief topics of conversation, it didn't seem a gloomy one at all. Sam, Dr. Schroeder assured us, was a super candidate.

"All we had to do was watch the way he put up with those tests," he said. "Lois Christopherson said he never batted an eye when she told him all the things he'd never be able to do again and what he'd have to put up with. He's just the kind of person we're looking for."

As Lois had done, he reviewed stage by stage the tortuous pilgrimage of the heart transplant. It was princely perils all over again. During the waiting period, we must understand that there were innumerable problems that could remove Sam from the transplant waiting list. An infection or a blood clot was automatic cause; even if a properly matched heart came along at that point, it would be useless to try to implant it.

If all went well and a heart was found for him, we must also understand that a very few recipients died on the operating table or suffered such physical incapacitation that recovery was impossible.

Dr. Schroeder emphasized, as had Lois, that the time spent in intensive care was the most hazardous. "Sam is virtually certain to have one or more severe rejections, possibly requiring removal and replacement of the first donor heart, and he will almost assuredly have one or two life-threatening infections. Both you and Sam have to be aware of these pitfalls. Here at Stanford we don't want anyone involved in this program to know anything less than the truth at all times. If Sam's sick, we'll tell you he is. If he's in danger of dying, you will be told. You will always know exactly where you stand, and there will be someone on call at the hospital twenty-four hours a day who is familiar with Sam's history, medicines, and exact present status."

I would never have expected that a doctor whose accents lay somewhere between a drawl and a twang could, with so few words and so little emotion, bestow such strength. It was like hearing, all at once, the Gettysburg Address, blood-sweat-and-tears, and "the only thing we have to fear is fear itself."

Totally unaware of his oratorical prowess, I'm sure, Dr. Schroeder handed Parker a list of telephone numbers. "If you are ever concerned about Sam during this waiting period or if you ever have a question about him, call us. Don't wait till morning; call on the spot. We're here."

I looked at Parker, as he held the list in his hand, and knew he was thinking with me that with the forces of Dr. Lincoln Churchill Roosevelt Schroeder behind us, Sam would never die by default. He would not just ebb out with the tide; if he did die, there would be a reason why he had to.

If all that was inspirational, what Dr. Schroeder said next was heady. Sam was Number One on the transplant list. No one else was waiting in line at the moment, and if a properly matched heart came along, it would be his. "Unless, of course," Dr. Schroeder added, "one of our present transplants gets in trouble and needs it. They're top priority."

We must never, therefore, be without or away from a telephone. If we left the place where we were living to go anywhere, Stanford wanted to know where. "If you go to the movies," Dr. Schroeder said, "give us the number of the theater. Be sure your phone is always in working order, and never, under any circumstances, do what one of our transplant candidates did: he moved to another apartment without telling us and missed his heart."

We didn't ask if the candidate ever had another chance; the story was too horrible even to contemplate. With Parker around, I knew such a thing would never happen to us.

Our last order was that Sam was to report every Thursday afternoon at one o'clock to the outpatient cardiac clinic to be checked over. This was essential.

We said good-bye, packed up Sam, and returned with him to the Holiday Inn. Parker's first act was to ring the desk, explain our situation, and ask to have our room phone tested. He could have saved himself the effort. Five minutes later Lois called. "Don't get excited," she said. "It's not a heart. I'm just checking to be sure we have your number right."

We didn't move to our new apartment until the next Thursday. The curtains, obedient to California law, didn't get cleaned until then, and although at home I am in charge of moves and housecleanings, Parker announced that in California he was. Every morning he departed for his housewifely chores at the apartment, leaving Sam and me to sit on our balcony at the Holiday Inn and gawk at the hotel visitors in the swimming pool beneath us. Parker had had our rooms switched to the sunny poolside of the hotel when Sam got out of the hospital. After watching a marvelously inebriated gentleman fall in fully clothed on the first afternoon, Sam and I couldn't have been more grateful to him. Anticipating another such disaster made the four-day wait quite bearable.

Daily Parker became more enraptured with his new nest. "Wait till you see it," he exulted to Sam and me. "Both bedrooms have huge windows, and the sun pours in all morning. There's even a little balcony, Sam, where you can catch the rays all day."

On Thursday we checked out of the Holiday Inn bag and baggage, went to clinic to hear with delight that Sam was still Number One on the transplant list, and drove to 1779 Woodland Avenue in Palo Alto, our new western headquarters. Stairs had become a nightmare for Sam — and for us who had to watch him climb them — and on Wednesday he had begun to complain that he had pulled a muscle in his back. That seemed odd, as he had done nothing even remotely athletic; but at any rate the elevator the apartment house boasted seemed heaven-sent. We gratefully packed Sam into it with our belongings and, walking up one flight, met him again at the top of the stairs.

Eyes shining with pride and importantly flourishing his keys, Parker undid both outside locks on the door of number 22 and flung it wide. "Look," he beamed. "Isn't this great?"

The one time I'd seen the apartment, while Sam was in the hospital, I'd noticed very little but the filthy gray wall-to-wall carpeting. That was certainly cleaner now, and if the windowless living room I gazed at was still a little gloomy, its walls were a lot whiter than they had been. Sam shuffled in ahead of me, took one look around, and collapsed on a worn but lengthy couch of uncertain vintage and doleful hue. Shades of dark olive with flecks of gold figured strongly in the apartment's decor, but Parker was waiting with such eager anticipation that I exclaimed, "Oh, darling, it's lovely! Don't you think so, Sam?"

"Yeah," he said from his new resting place, without much enthusiasm. "Kinda plastic, though, isn't it?" And "the plastic apartment" it became from that moment on.

That night, for the first time, we were forced to leave Sam alone — for an hour, while Parker drove me to the airport. It made us both very nervous. It was December 9, and I was to fly home on the night plane — ominously referred to by the travel agent who booked me on it as the "red-eye special" — leaving Parker to tend Sam. I would return to California on the twenty-first to take over for three weeks, and Parker would go back to Maine. We had abandoned the idea of Christmas together the minute I saw the California pansies. "It won't be like Christmas anyway with all those foolish flowers," I had said to Parker. "It would be crazy for you to come out just for two days," and he had agreed. With our three-week plan, one of us would always be with Sam, and Alix would never suffer for lack of a parent for more than forty-eight hours.

Pristine in my now stain-free traveling off-white when we arrived at the apartment about three, by seven, when we drove up the freeway to the airport, I was a disgrace all over again. Parker's nesting instincts had not drawn him to bureau drawers, kitchen cupboards, or closet floors, and I had spent four hours on all fours, cleaning out the residue of the former tenants, who appeared to have had copious amounts of black hair and bizarre sexual appetites. The how-to-do-it book I found in the bureau in Sam's room bore little resemblance to the how-to-do-it books of my acquaintance, and the hooded orange light bulb hovering at a most extraordinary height over the plastic top of the dining-room table could only lead me to believe that how you did it was there. It boggled the mind.

I cried all the way to the airport, which distressed Parker. "Don't, Vic," he kept saying, because he hates despair, and I tried to stop, but I couldn't. I had loved Parker for so long. With him, nothing in all our years together had seemed insurmountable. But I suddenly realized on the way to my plane that I was going to be on one coast or the other without him until Sam either lived or died, and I didn't know how I could bear it.

Chapter Eight
I cried, missing Sam and Parker, all the way home and repeated my ocean-to-ocean weep-in in honor of the other children twelve days later when I went back to California. Happily for my dignity neither plane was full, and I managed to snivel away with a modicum of decorum and an empty seat beside me, but in truth, had the planes been booked solid, I don't think I could have stopped.

The time in Maine was pure Charles Dickens in being simultaneously the best and the worst of times. The worst began the very night I got home. Parker called to say that Sam was back in the hospital. The pain in his back had not been a pulled muscle; it was a blood clot in his lung, and he was off the transplant waiting list indefinitely.

I knew just enough about blood clots to be in panic. "I'll come right back out," I said, but Parker was adamant.

"No," he said, "you can't. Sam's pretty miserable right now, but Dr. Schroeder says clots do clear up — sometimes even in a week or so. He's got him on all kinds of medication with IVs and the whole works, and your coming out here wouldn't accomplish anything. I'm here, and Alix needs you there. The only way we're going to make this damn thing work is to divide up."

He was right, and I didn't protest, but for the first time I sensed that holding up the Maine end of Sam's ordeal could be even worse than coping in California. At least there, however bad things were, you were a part of them.

"He took all the needles and the tubes without a word," Parker said, "but, God, it just killed me to see the look in his eyes when they said he was off the list. It's an awful setback for him when he was so ready to go for the heart. The poor kid's just hanging on the ropes, and the worst of it is, he's lost his place. There were two other guys behind him, an O Negative and an O Positive, and they're Number One and Two now."

Parker sounded so sunk I only told him that Tina was home from England, Malcolm was out of the Coast Guard for good, and he and Ruthie were all moved in with us. I didn't tell him that, home less than six hours, I had already backed his car into a tree on my way to pick up Tina at the airport.

I also avoided telling him that the new part of the house which we needed for the Christmas throngs was nowhere near finished and that our new bathtub had been inadvertently installed with mortuary-gray tiles.

The best of times were just being home with the others again. I walked with Moriah and skated with the children. Ruthie was completely off balance with her new shape, and Alix and Tina or Malcolm and Charlie had to take turns supporting her around the pond. Laughing and shivering with cold, we'd all walk back to the house, singing off-key Christmas carols, to be joined for supper by Pokie, the only currently employed Poole.

The days were no problem. There was so much to do and so many people to contend with, there wasn't time to worry. By the time breakfast was over for some, it was lunchtime for others, and what was it I'd planned for dinner? In between meals Tina and Ruthie and I decorated the house and Alix wrapped presents, while Dottie valiantly baked pies and Christmas cookies amid the chaos, and Malcolm and Charlie beat strategic daily retreats to Malcolm's new house to escape us. It was only after they succeeded in procuring, in their father's absence, the first symmetrical Christmas tree the Poole family had ever had that they redeemed themselves in the eyes of the ladies.

Having the children around me was an escape from reality, and only when I got into bed at night did the horrors come crowding in again. I knew I had to go back to California, and I wanted to be with Sam for Christmas more than anything in the world, but I couldn't imagine how I would possibly make myself pack, walk out the door, and say good-bye to the other children.

Tina was to drive me to the airport, and when the day came I did pack at five in the morning, I did walk out the door at six thirty, and I kissed the others and hugged them, but I couldn't say good-bye. It was snowing and sleeting. I took one last look at the doorway — where Malcolm and Charlie and Ruthie, with her arms around Alix, stood waving at me — and stumbled to the car behind Tina, with my head down and my eyes blinded by tears that didn't stop for thirty-five hundred miles.

When I got to San Francisco, my luggage hadn't, and there was no Parker to meet me. Grief turned to panic. Sam had gotten out of the hospital the day before, but he still had the blood clot, and I was sure that something awful had happened to him. I waited on the curb outside the airport for more than an hour and then called the plastic apartment.

"H'lo," said Sam drearily.

"It's me, your mother," I said. "Where's Daddy?" I wished I hadn't asked because the next voice I heard was Parker's and it was infuriated.

"What the hell's going on?" he demanded. "Ruth called and said there was a storm and you'd missed your Boston connection."

"But I didn't," I protested. "I'm here, and I've lost my luggage and all Sam's Christmas presents, and why are you mad at me?"

That did nothing to placate him, but we finally agreed that I would wait till the next plane came in from the East in an hour, in hopes that the baggage was on it, and he would pick me up then.

Waiting seemed vastly preferable to confronting an irate Parker, and I went back through the gate of the baggage area. It was empty of people, it was empty of luggage, it was empty of any place to sit, and when I tried to get back through the gate, it had locked.

"Shit," I said in refined New Englandese, and, noticing a line of phone booths on the wall, I retreated to one to sit out my despair on its little corner perch. I suddenly realized as I sat down that I was not alone. Over the glass wall of the booth, I could see another despairing form. A large gentleman was sitting on the corner perch of the adjoining phone booth with his head in his hands. It seemed odd because he appeared to be an airline employee. He was wearing an official-looking parka with a badge with his picture on it, and I was just trying to screw up my courage to ask him how I could get out when he stood up, tore across the room to a door marked POSITIVELY NO EXIT, and exited.

I went after him, but when I started out POSITIVELY NO EXIT, the most terrible clamor of bells and alarms went off. Every doorway leading to the baggage area suddenly filled with faces, and uniformed guards rushed to the fences and gates surrounding me, as I stood there quaking, hat in hand, in my doomed traveling off-white.

They did let me out with the utmost scorn, but Parker couldn't have cared less about my adventure when I finally found both him and the luggage.

"Ruth said you missed the plane," he snarled as he hurled the suitcases in the back seat of the car.

"But why is it my fault? Why are you mad at *me*?" I argued.

"I hate changes of plan," said this entirely new Parker that I didn't think I was going to like at all. "And stop crying, for Christ's sake. You cried all the way up to the airport when you went home and you're still crying. Can't you think of anything else to do?"

He was so totally unfair that I stopped in mid-sob. "I am crying," I said with icy self-control, "because I have left my children and because I am not going to be with them for Christmas, and, yes, I can think of something else to do. I can think of a whole list of names to call you, beginning with *bastard*," and we drove the rest of the way to the plastic apartment in stony silence.

Standing with pursed lips waiting for Parker to fumble the keys to the building out of his pocket, I could find nothing encouraging in my new surroundings. It was the year of the drought, and gray dust covered the leaves of the few sparse bushes set in earth baked hard as clay. Gum wrappers lay disconsolately amid the shrubbery, and through the glass facade that formed the front of our building I could see the vivid blue and black-flocked paper that covered the walls of the two-story stairwell. It was even more repulsive than I had remembered, and I turned my head away to regard instead the side of the building, which was entirely preoccupied with balconies.

Ours was the corner one on the second floor, just to the left of the glass facade, and it now boasted — which it hadn't when I left — a huge shade umbrella, stuck crookedly in the center of a rusty-legged table. Apparently at some point the umbrella had been white with orange flowers, but it was no longer, and the large pussycat sitting on the railing of the balcony below ours was meowing dismally, as if he liked his environment as little as I did.

Following an equally lip-pursed Parker through the cabbage-laden odors of the hallway, past the threadbare aqua and gilt-flecked reception couch, and up the stairs, I tried to avoid looking at the wallpaper. There was another pocket-fumbling outside our apartment, and I was standing there feeling as if the world were coming to an end when Parker opened the door.

Against the white wall inside, to the left of the door, I saw a little Christmas tree that had to be real because I could smell it. I saw carefully arranged Christmas cards everywhere, a huge bunch of real holly on the plastic top of the dining-room table, and there was Sam, turning his head toward the door from the olive and gold-flecked sofa to see who was coming in. Call it a moment of truth or whatever, but in that split second when Parker opened the door, rage, anguish, and homesickness all vanished. Standing in the doorway, I knew that unless we had this awful Christmas, we could never have a happy one again. We were more together now, divided though we were, than we could ever be at home without Sam, and all at once I knew that I could have said good-bye to the other children with a hug and a smile and a wave. After I'd kissed Sam, I turned to Parker and said, "Well, you can delete *bastard*."

Parker's tree was his triumph. Lacking proper ornaments, he had trimmed it with matchbooks and gum wrappers, Sam's plastic wristband from the hospital, and tickets from the hospital parking lot.

My triumph was the six-o'clock news heard on the TV he had rented for Sam. "An armed airline employee this afternoon attempted to hijack a seven-forty-seven jetliner at San Francisco International Airport," announced the newscaster, and there on the screen was my baggage-room companion, his uniform parka and badge augmented now by handcuffs.

It was good not to feel torn between my two families anymore, but there was little comfort in looking at Sam. He was even bluer and quieter and thinner, and he coughed endlessly. The fact that Parker and I now finally understood, thanks to Stanford's evaluation of his condition, that the cough was caused by failing lungs didn't make it any easier to listen to. We gave up trying to sleep and were on our third cup of coffee by seven o'clock the next morning; Parker was leaving for Portland that night, and we tried to catch up on everything that had happened since we were last together or that might happen before we were together again.

I wasn't imagining that the cough was worse since the blood clot. "Thank God, we got him out here when we did," Parker said. "They'd never have accepted him if the clot had come a week earlier. I only hope to hell it clears up soon and he can get back on the list, because I know, once he gets a chance at a heart, he'll make it. He wants it so. You should have seen him when we met the guy who'd gotten a transplant a year ago. He just lit up."

Parker had told me over the phone before I came back about that man. He was at Stanford for his annual checkup and had told Sam that before his transplant he hadn't been able to even lift a pound. He was now lifting hundred-pound weights.

"He was a great big healthy-looking guy," he said. "You wouldn't think he'd been sick a day in his life."

Clinic was a day early because of Christmas, but when we took Sam there that afternoon, the thought of his ever lifting weights seemed absurd. It was all he could do to pick up his feet. Parker and I sat together at one end of the long passageway that formed the clinic waiting room while Sam shuffled off down to the other end toward the labs for his blood work and X-rays.

"I didn't remember that the hall was so long the first time we brought him here," I said. Parker's answer brought me little consolation.

"I didn't either," he said. "I think it's because he's walking so slowly."

A thoroughly modern mother was sitting next to us, loudly explaining to her child that there was no Santa Claus and "no Easter Bunny either," and I had to sit on both my hands to keep from reaching over and slapping her.

As I drove him to the airport that night, Parker gave me my orders. I was to be sure the doors and windows were locked every night, I was not to go anywhere near the Laundromat after dark (two blocks away, it was on a street referred to by one and all as Whiskey Gulch), I was to start the car every day, and the way I was to park it in the garage under the plastic apartment was "carefully." Tearless, to his delight, I kissed him good-bye and drove back down the freeway to Sam and to Christmas, marveling at the tenant who had dared to leave the following message on Parker's windshield:

Dear Person,

Who the fuck do you think you are parking in two places neither of which is yours. Further transgressions of this reprehensible nature, and the next note will be attached to a brick.

Signed:
Warmly

Parker had sheepishly pulled it out of his pocket and handed it to me when we got to the terminal.

When I got back to the apartment, however, it was apparent that it was not I who was to become the new head of the California branch of Pooles. It was Sam who locked the doors and checked the windows, and only the bittersweet answer he gave me when I thanked him for making me feel so protected made me realize how vulnerable he felt. "Great," he said, "till we get a burglar. A hell of a lot of help I'd be. I'd fall down if he touched me."

By Christmas Eve Sam and I had established a daily routine that seemed quite endurable to me as long as I had him to endure it with, and to my complete surprise I found myself liking "the plastic." Parker had done wonders for it while I'd been gone. The landlady had originally given us two blankets, but Parker had prevailed upon her sympathies with Sam's perpetually congealed state, and she had produced two more. Sam used three. On our bed was a fire-engine-red fuzzy cover that needed no label to state that it was manufactured from man-made material; it was the synthetic to end all synthetics. It smelled dreadful and it not only felt dreadful, it felt like nothing I have ever touched before. It slipped and caught simultaneously, but it was gloriously warm. He had also acquired three new sheets and several new towels, and our kitchen now afforded two glass glasses along with its five plastic ones. We had three large plastic dinner plates, several smaller ones, and two cereal bowls of matching design. We had two saucepans, a frying pan, a spatula with a broken handle, and two china coffee mugs, one of which had SAM printed on it. It was all we needed, and the apartment was all we needed too.

The one glass wall of each bedroom faced the one glass wall of a room in the identical building next to us. If I ever forgot to pull the curtain when I went to sleep at night, I would sit up in bed and stretch in the morning to see my neighbor across the alley sitting up and stretching in his. If he'd promptly leapt up in mortification as I did to avoid being viewed, he would have rushed headlong out the bedroom door into a long narrow hall. There he would have had a choice; he could either have closeted himself at one end in the windowless bathroom, which grew mold at an alarming rate, or he could have fled in the other direction, past the second bedroom, to enter the daytime quarters — the living room, dining room, and kitchen. It was really all one big room, and furniture, not walls, divided it into its proper segments.

The living room was Sam's world. It held his sofa, a matching chair, and the TV. It also afforded two plastic-topped end tables, a coffee table, and another huge imitation leather chair which I avoided sitting in because putting a hand down either side of the seat produced old cigarette butts, wads of chewed gum, or worse.

The dining-room table was my world, and it, with its four black wrought-iron chairs with olive and gold-flecked plastic seats and backs, comprised the dining room. Parker had raised the hooded shade above it and replaced the orange bulb. The table having become properly asexual again, I could attend to Sam's sofa world from it and fetch him what he needed from the kitchen section of the room behind it. At it I wrote, and read, and did my needlepoint, or gazed through the glass doors in front of it at Parker's new umbrella table on the balcony outside.

It was a strange life for someone used to running up and down stairs from six in the morning until ten at night. The oven in the stove never did work, but that was a small matter because, except for a grape popsicle, a scrambled egg, or maybe a little cereal, Sam didn't eat anyway.

Other than five- or ten-minutes' conversation at night, he didn't talk either. He would say, "Ice, please," or "C'n I have another cup?" which meant that his spit cup was filled again with blood and mucus, but the rest of the time he lay silent and remote, huddled under his blankets on the sofa, his eyes focused somewhere on the wall above the television set.

He turned the TV on the minute he came into the room in the morning, declining to read or be read to. From my world at the table, I couldn't see the screen, and although I am not a television watcher, sometimes I'd hear something that piqued my curiosity. "Who said that?" I'd say, or, "What happened?" and he'd always say, "I dunno." I couldn't understand why, and I never said anything to him, but it bothered me.

I learned to make myself stay away from the bathroom when I heard him gagging and choking his way through his morning shower that now truly did last an hour. With the drought it was evil to waste water, but I didn't care. It was only in the shower, Sam told me, that he was ever warm or that he could breathe without hurting. Since it was impossible to concentrate on anything else while the terrible noises were coming from the bathroom, I'd put down my book and pick up my needlepoint, jabbing the needle fiercely in and out of the mesh to keep myself from jumping up at every retch and groan.

I learned that when he asked for cereal in the morning or an egg at night, it meant that he felt nauseated and wanted to vomit. "It doesn't hurt so much when you have something in your stomach to throw up," he explained, and after I gave him the food, I would get a wet washcloth ready to hold on his head.

There was so little I could do to make him happy that it became essential that I do nothing to make him unhappy. If happiness was a dry towel, or a smooth bed, or a grape popsicle, he should have them, and if unhappiness was listening to a vacuum cleaner, then it was better to be dirty.

I learned that a bright spot in his day was at two thirty when the mail came, and I would rush downstairs to the mailbox, blessing the residents of Kent School and Greater Portland who kept it full.

A bright spot in my day was my afternoon walk to the store for his paper, and it was another one for Sam too because it gave him his only privacy. Invariably when I came back he would be a little perkier, saying, "I just talked to Fred. His mother says hi," or, "Was it okay for me to call Brad in Philadelphia? He's home from Kent for vacation."

"Be my guest," I'd say, "it's only money," but it wasn't only money. The telephone seemed to have become his lifeline, and the brightest spot in both our days was the telephone call home — and until after Christmas we called or were called daily.

He'd talk to Parker and anyone else who was around with yups and okays and then at the end he'd say, "Lemme talk to Al," and for the few seconds he did he was Sam again.

"Why doncha come on out here for Christmas, Al? I've got a big double bed. You can share it with me."

I could hear Alix squealing indignantly, "I wouldn't sleep with you for a million dollars, Sam!" and Sam would say, "Hell, Al, I'd sleep with anybody for a million dollars," and after we'd hung up he'd say, "She misses me, you know."

The worst part of the day was after we'd gone to bed. I'd hear him coughing in the next room or, even worse, I'd not hear him coughing and wonder if he was still alive. Knowing that he very well might not be made the nights unbearable. I'd try to concentrate on the letter my cousin Bill Scott had written us from Vanderbilt: "I hope all of you have the best possible Christmas under the circumstances and I think you are going to have a good one because you have made a faithful decision to do a very proper thing."

It will be a good one, I'd tell myself, but, being me, more often than not I'd start remembering instead the article he had enclosed, "Rehabilitation after Cardiac Transplantation," by Lois Christopherson. It was very optimistic about "after," but Sam was off the transplant list and the article said: "All but two of thirty-two patients selected for but not recipients of a transplant died within twenty-one weeks of the time of official acceptance." I'd figured it out on the homemade calendar I'd drawn up the day after I came back to California; twenty-one weeks from December 3 was April 29. That didn't make it any easier to go to sleep.

The funny thing was that in a way Bill Scott was right, and parts of Christmas, thanks to Sam, were wonderful, but it didn't start out that way. Christmas Eve fell on a Friday that year, and the day began with Sam talking, which made it different from any other we'd spent together. He announced that he thought we should have clams and lobsters for Christmas dinner and that I should find some.

It seemed a strange choice of menu for someone who had consumed one grape popsicle, two mouthfuls of cereal, and half an egg in two days, but I started off on my quest. I'm a terrible driver in strange places; I can't see street signs or route signs, but I had to go alone because Sam said sitting in the car hurt too much.

I found the clams and lobsters at a fish market, but I couldn't find my way back to the apartment. Three times by mistake I got on the freeway heading south, and three times with mounting panic I pictured Sam abandoned and dying in the apartment. I was a basket case when I finally did get back, but Sam was disgusted with me when I said I was never going to drive anywhere again other than to clinic or the airport. I had to get mellow, he said.

It wasn't mellow I felt when I set off on my afternoon walk to get his newspaper, and after I'd seen the Christmas lights twinkling in every window and the fathers coming home early from work, what I felt was miserable. I'd promised myself I wouldn't think about home, but I couldn't help it. With the time change, everyone would be at Bill and Rozzie's Christmas Eve party by now — dogs and children and friends, eggnog and cheese fondue, Christmas greens, and a confusion of presents. I wondered, when the party was over and they'd gotten back to our house, if Tina and Ruthie would remember where I'd left the Christmas stockings. I wondered who'd read "the night before Christmas" with me not there, or if they'd read it at all, and I inelegantly swiped at my nose with a gloved hand.

"Oh, God, 'I am not Prince Hamlet, nor was meant to be,'" I sniveled, going down one street. "What the hell am I doing in a mess like this?" And going up another, I tried to pull myself together with an old school motto, "Do it with thy might," but it didn't help at all.

I even tried, as I'd tried since Sam got sick, to pray, but that didn't work either. The Episcopal church at home had long since shattered Rozzie's and my direct pipeline to the Lord. "Never turn your back on the Church, girls," Mother had always cautioned us; "you will need it." But her loyalty was evidently not part of a reciprocal-trade agreement with our church. The last Sunday morning she was well enough to attend services was almost the last she saw of the clergy, and the rector of our church had not only been late for *her* funeral, he had had to be urged from his office by the children for Daddy's. Every time I tried to hear the "comfortable words our Saviour Christ saith," I heard instead the most uncomfortable words of the rector of our church — "I don't like to get to burial services too early. It's a waste of time" — and they interfered with God and me.

The clerk at the store where I bought the paper had changed his usual "Have a nice day" to "Have a nice Christmas," and I started home feeling even more wretched and abandoned. It seemed so strange that I who read ends of books before beginnings, who watched movies through separated fingers, who hated change, should be involved in desperate matters and far from home on Christmas Eve.

"I bet Jesus was born on a Wednesday too," I told myself, thinking of poor old Sam on his sofa and finding the logic soothing; and I plodded along, trying to ignore the father at one house who was trying to smuggle a shiny new bicycle into his garage. At Bill and Rozzie's by now, Parker would be saying, "Okay, all you shock troops. Time to move 'em out. We've got a lot to do tonight." It might even be snowing in Maine. I could see Parker and the children, piling out of the cars at our house, laughing and running through the snowflakes to the back door, with Moriah at their heels, and I felt as if my heart were breaking.

When I got to the street that ran into ours, though, the Lord must have taken pity on me and my tears. Tactfully bypassing our Episcopal church, and moving in one of his mysterious ways, he sent me a Christmas present. Suddenly I could hear the voice of a friend who had escaped from the Nazis, as clearly as though he were walking along beside me. I'd complained to him once that I felt inadequate, and he'd laughed at me.

"If you can control what you can touch with one arm outstretched, Vicky, you're doing a good job," he'd said, and, right there on the corner of Newell Street, I knew that that was what I was trying to do. I was trying to do a good job, and if his words weren't as imposing as "Do it with thy might," they were much better suited to me; I wasn't very imposing either.

I looked at the dead brown leaves falling on rosebushes in full bloom and thought, Well, it really isn't like Christmas out here anyway, and I was humming "Good Christian men, rejoice" as I marched over the little bridge that separated our street from its more affluent neighbors. The dry ravine beneath it was as depressing as ever, but I felt fine, and every time the carol came to "give ye heed to what we say," I sang "car-di-o-my-o-pa-thy" instead. It was very satisfying.

My second Christmas present from the Lord was Sam. When I got back to the apartment, he was on the crest of the wave. We talked on the telephone until ten, and until ten thirty we opened the stockings that Tina had filled for us, which made me very nervous because it was only Christmas Eve. Sam said, however, that it was good this year to do things differently, and that, "thanks a bunch," I didn't have to recite "the night before Christmas" either.

Instead he recited his vices of the past. I learned for a fact that he'd started smoking in the fifth grade — "only from time to time" — which I'd suspected, and drunk beer in the ninth, which Dottie had told me about, but "pot in the tenth?"

"Fred's mother caught us out in the backyard. God, was she mad!"

But that was only a beginning. By the time he'd catalogued the trip to Florida and his night forays of the summer, I was a broken woman. "Dear God," I said. "No wonder you're sick!"

He'd been lying on his back, regarding the ceiling as he reviewed his shady past, but when he heard what I said, he rolled over. "I don't care," he said. "I'd rather be dead than be a vegetable. Like I told you, I wouldn't give up anything I've ever done. We've had an awful lot of fun — our family — Mum, haven't we?" So I learned that he loved us.

I learned that he wanted new ski boots for Christmas next year, and I learned that he knew he was needed. "Everybody takes things too seriously without me. Hell, I bet Pokie won't even go on the ice run and count drunks without me there," he said. Above all, I learned what Kent meant to him.

"The fall before I got sick," he said, "I think I knew I was. Sometimes playing football it hurt so to breathe and I'd cough all the time, but I'd just keep playing like I had to, you know. That's why I guess I was so up about that varsity letter; I guess I knew I'd never have another chance at it, and I really wanted it. It's just the same now about going back to Kent. I started it, and I'm going to keep going and going, and I'm going to graduate. It's all I want."

"You will," I said. "I know you will," and I walked over to my homemade calendar. "Look, your next clinic is December thirtieth; you'll get back on the list then. Give them a week to decide the clot's really gone and round up a heart, and that's January sixth. The next day will be your heart day — January seventh. I can feel it inside."

Louise skied ten miles that night through the wilds of Wyoming, where she was an instructor for a wilderness expedition, to get to a telephone so she could call Sam. "Tell Joe he's incredible, Aunt Vic," she said to me when she hung up. "He is, you know."

"Well, not average," I said. "That's for sure."

I was writing Parker at my table the next morning when I heard a Christmas carol, and, although it was still dawn by his standards, Sam emerged from his room carrying the FM stereo radio Parker had given him before he left.

"Merry Christmas, Mum," he said. "Gotta have a little Christmas mood music, y'know," and he came over to the table and kissed me.

He was a ludicrous sight. His underdrawers hung wide on either side of his long bony legs, and I looked up at him, grayish blue and skeletal, and just shook my head. "Merry Christmas, darling," I said. "You *are* incredible, and I love you!"

He gave me a book for Christmas, and when I asked him how he'd ever managed to go Christmas shopping, he was insulted. "Gawd, Mum, I always do my Christmas shopping. Charlie took me the Saturday before we came out here. It hurt like hell and Charlie had to carry everything, but I got presents for everybody" — and the calls from home confirmed that he had.

We talked again to everyone we knew that Christmas Day. We ate the California lobsters and the California clams, but at three thirty our revels ended. The effort of giving me a merry Christmas — of being for me what Malcolm had solemnly pronounced him at birth, "an everlasting Christmas present" — almost finished Sam. Without warning a migraine struck with all its attendant woes, and when I finally got him out of the bathroom and into bed, he was as cold as death and soaking wet with icy perspiration. I sat on the edge of his bed near the window for hours that night, watching the family in the apartment opposite ours eat their Christmas dinner at their bright yellow table with its bright yellow chairs, oddly enough feeling no emotion at all.

The next morning, however, when I passed his door, he was lying across the bed as if he'd fallen there. His feet were still on the floor, but his head was thrown back and his eyes were open. Daddy had been found in exactly the same position the morning that he died, and it was déjà vu of the most terrible kind. Even though Sam started to cough almost immediately, I was shattered, but during the morning I made a decision that for some strange reason comforted me. If Sam did die in the apartment, I was going to call Parker and tell him. After that, regardless of what he told me to do, I was going to do nothing until he got to California. I was going to sit with Sam as I had sat with Daddy, waiting for Rozzie to get in town from the Cape, and no one was going to touch him until we were both together with him.

Day by long day, the holidays passed. The receptionist at

the clinic had been told about us by a friend of a friend in the East, and she would call and say, "Everything okay? You know where I live if you get lonely," and I loved her for leaving it up to us because there were those who didn't. The McDuffys, for instance. Who were the McDuffys? No one knew, but they had our names, and they wanted to visit us. Parker and Sam and I had managed to keep them at bay over the telephone, but they finally appeared at the door of our apartment one afternoon just after Christmas, bearing gifts.

I didn't offer them chairs, and they sat down. I didn't say anything, and they talked.

Mrs. McDuffy turned her attentions first to Sam. "My daughter is a candy striper on the pediatric floor where you'll be, dear," she said. "You'll just love her."

It should have been evident to Mrs. McDuffy, from the expression on his face, that her daughter would not love Sam. To his credit, though, he only said, "I won't be on the pediatric floor."

"Oh, yes, you will, dear," she said firmly. "All the children are there!"

Sam demolished, she turned her attentions to me.

"Our church group loves to get involved with people who are troubled. How many people do you know in the area, Mrs. Poole, that you can turn to?"

"None," I said. "I-like-to-be-alone," and the McDuffys departed. We never saw them again, but I ate the Christmas cookies she brought, and they were delicious.

When I came back from my walk that afternoon, Sam was in tears. "I'm so tired of hurting everywhere," he said. "I'm so tired of being cold all the time and being sick. I'm so tired of waiting."

I remember him laughing just once after that. Craig

Clark, the boy he'd painted with the summer before, came to spend the night with us, bearing in his arms a huge box. When Sam unwrapped it, I couldn't believe my eyes. It was a child's toy. There was a building, as I remember, and dozens of little wooden figures.

Sam really did laugh for a second, and as I stared blankly Craig said, "It's the Weebles, Mrs. Poole. It's how I got Sam home all last summer when he couldn't walk," and he tried to tip over one of the little figurines, which wiggled and rolled about but refused to collapse.

"See?" he said. " 'Weebles wobble, but they don't fall down.' That's what I kept saying to Sam. I'd hold him up on one side and yell that at him, and he always made it."

It was good to hear Sam laugh, but to this day the Weebles aren't funny to me, and after Craig left nothing could even be remotely construed as amusing. Sam didn't get back on the list on December 30, as I'd prophesied he would.

"I can still hear the rattle," Dr. Schroeder said, "and I can still see the clot on the X-ray. It's getting smaller, but he can't go back on the list yet."

Napoleon's retreat from Moscow couldn't have taken any longer or been any more depressing than was ours from the clinic to the plastic apartment. Napoleon at least had a future to plan for, even if it was only Waterloo, and an army to worry about. Poor old Sam had only me.

Good soldier to the end, though, he turned defeat into an assault and ordered me, the army of one, with unwavering authority. He cursed the cars that stopped in the city center to park and me for not accelerating to sixty between lights.

"Goddamned jaywalkers," he snarled as I stopped to let

a child cross the street, but when we got home he lay on the sofa with such despair on his face that I wanted to run to him and throw my arms around him, but I knew it would only make things worse.

"Look," I said fiercely, pointing to January 7 on my calendar. "I told you you'd get your heart then. You have a whole eight days to get over the clot," but the coming seven days before the next clinic stretched ahead of us like the Sahara.

At least, though, my attack got him talking again. He rolled over on the sofa later on and said, "If I do get a heart, I'll be susceptible to diabetes, gangrene, and bone dissolution for the rest of my life," which I expect was an improvement over the silence.

I was glad to see New Year's come and I was even gladder to see it go. Children set off firecrackers under our windows all day on New Year's Eve, and the pussycat below us, abandoned for the weekend, howled mournfully for attention. Sam was annoyed beyond belief by the time we settled down to watch 1976 depart on TV. The only thing I remember him saying all night was, "Do you think there are any parents who wouldn't do this for their kid?" And when I said I couldn't imagine any, he sat up and looked at me, and without hostility, but with the utmost authority, he said, "You know you and Dad would have been murderers if you hadn't let me do this."

The full feeling had been plaguing him all day, and after he said that he went to bed, leaving me shaking at the idea that if we hadn't brought him to Stanford, he would have died at home thinking that.

My shaking continued till dawn, but after midnight it was courtesy of five earth tremors that rocked Palo Alto, and I quaked sleepless along with them until I heard Sam call me from the bathroom. He had been throwing up, and he just pointed to the toilet; it was filled with blood.

"I bled when I went to the bathroom too," he said, "but I'm not going back to the hospital. I don't want to be in there again."

Thinking back on that morning, I didn't act like me at all. "It's probably nothing at all," I said, in the most down-to-earth manner, "and if you go to Emergency and get it checked out, I'm sure we'll be back in time for the football game. If you don't," I warned with an authority I didn't feel, "it will surely get worse. I know all about bleeding." And to my amazement he got his pants and sweater on, and we went to the hospital.

Even more to my amazement, I was right. The dosage of blood thinner he was taking was too high and his clotting time too long. It was a good thing that we had come to the hospital before it got out of hand, they said, and we were indeed back in the apartment in time for the game, another half day closer to clinic.

I didn't dare go for a walk that afternoon with Sam's medicines out of whack, but the events of the morning had certainly jaundiced my disposition. I wrote to Tina that I couldn't imagine why anyone would want to go outdoors in California anyway.

"How nauseating," I remarked, "are the flora and fauna. The fauna are bad enough, and are cats, all loathsome and everywhere, and tied-up dogs with coats that are never one color but hundreds of mottled effects; but the flora are worse. Great obscene things with red insides hang on every tree in the most disgusting shapes and fall on my proper New England head whenever I walk, and a trip to the supermarket leaves me feeling that I have been to an X-rated movie. Dreadful place! I like acorns, and pine cones, and berries."

Nothing is worse than feeling dismal when the rest of the world is whooping it up, and it was a great relief when the holidays were behind us. Suddenly I woke up one morning thinking, My God, clinic is only day after tomorrow — we're actually getting through the week. And to make things even better, Lynn Honma (with hope, Sam's future nurse) came to visit. She had come to see Sam and Parker when Sam was in the hospital with his blood clot, and she was just as much fun and as pretty as they had told me. She was tiny — about five feet one — with brown, almond-shaped eyes that actually danced and short, dark, wavy hair, but the Christmas present she gave us would have compensated for the appearance of a Gorgon. It was a Hawaiian calendar that her parents had sent her, and I expect that it was a measure of the bleakness of our lives that I was genuinely ecstatic at the thought of being able to dispense with my own homemade effort. If Lynn thought my appreciation unbalanced, she didn't show it then, and when she left she gave me a hug and said, "I liked Parker and Sam so much that I knew I'd like you too, and I do."

My day was made, and I spent the rest of it going over in my mind everything she had told us. From Lois we had learned the practicalities of getting a heart transplant and from Dr. Schroeder the medical intricacies, but it was Lynn who filled us in on the human-relations end, and it was through her that I finally understood how a heart got from the donor to the recipient. In California it was not preserved in solution and then palpated to start beating again, as Dr. Bushman, the psychiatrist we had seen in Portland, had surmised; it was in most cases directly removed from the donor in one operating room, rushed next door to another, and plunked into the already open chest of the recipient.

"In California," Lynn had explained, "there is a brain-death law, and it's usually from brain-death cases that our donor hearts come."

I had gulped and swallowed and said nothing then, but after Lynn left I couldn't stop thinking about it. "God," I'd said to Sam. "I guess it hardly misses a beat," and my respect for donor families increased a hundredfold.

Lynn had explained to us how Sam would look after the operation. "He'll still be hooked up to the respirator," she said, "and there will be a huge tube in his mouth when he comes back from the operating room and more tubes in his nose, and catheters in his bladder and tubes in his chest. There will be a tube in a vein in his neck, and all his medications will be given through that at the beginning. You'll probably see all the equipment and say, 'Oh, my God, what have they done to him?' " but I was not to be nervous.

"I'll be there," she said, "and my best friend is going to help me. We'll be busy, but you just feel Sam's feet. He'll be all pink and white, and the next day he'll probably be sitting up in a chair and so bossy you'll wish he were sick again."

It had become quite clear while we talked to Lynn that Sam had picked up founts of heretofore unmentioned information at clinic, for when he asked her about the two transplants who were currently in ICU, he called them by name.

Lynn started to giggle when he said, "How's Cobbie

doing?" Cobbie, she said, was sneaking beer, and all the doctors were currently cross with him, but she didn't smile when he asked her about Burpee, the other. He'd had a setback and wasn't doing well at all.

"You know, though," she said after that, "there's always some reason, Sam, why something goes wrong. Burpee's a wonderful man and he's trying hard, but he's a lot older, and that makes it harder."

There it was again; Sam would never die by default, and that thought kept me going all afternoon in the soap-opera silence of the plastic apartment. Lynn had invited me to tour the intensive care unit with her on the next clinic day while Sam was having his tests, and, although my first reaction was that the ICU was the last thing I wanted to see until I had to, after she left I found myself actually looking forward to my visit.

Before clinic time could roll around again, though, Rozzie called. "I took one look at Parker's face on New Year's Eve," she said. "I never saw anyone look so worried and miserable in my life. I'm coming out," and she didn't have to bring up any otherworldly discussion she'd had with Mother on the matter. I needed her.

Auntie Mame from head to foot in fox-collared ultrasuede and wide-brimmed burgundy hat, and with me trailing in her wake, she swept upstairs — oblivious to the odors of cabbage, to the decadent condition of the reception couch, and even to the blue and black-flocked wallpaper — and into the plastic apartment.

To our joint surprise, Sam was sitting up on his sofa as if he were quite himself, entertaining a Kent friend of Tina's and Charlie's who lived nearby.

"I came," Rozzie hissed indignantly after she had removed her coat and followed me into the kitchen, "because you and Parker said that Sam was too sick to talk or even sit up. What do you call what he's doing now?"

"Making an effort," I said. "Wait till she leaves." And no sooner had the friend departed than he said, "Glad you're here, Aunt Roz, but I feel kind of sick," and repaired to the bathroom to begin a vomiting bout that was still going on when we went to clinic the next day.

Rozzie went with us, and, while Sam had his tests, Lynn took us on the promised tour of ICU and even introduced us to Dr. Shumway. Neither institution appeared to be in the least formidable, but both seemed far removed from Sam's needs when we found him after clinic.

He didn't speak till we got to the car. "The other O Negative who took my place is getting his heart tomorrow," he said, "and the O Positive who was waiting is dead," and it wasn't till I asked about the clot that he told me he was finally, after almost a month, back on the waiting list.

When we got to the apartment he started vomiting again, and there was no satisfaction in looking at Lynn's calendar and seeing that tomorrow was January 7. I'd been right — it was going to be a heart day, but not Sam's.

Rozzie was as desperate as Parker and I by the time she went home. "I'd never have understood if I hadn't come," she said, when she hugged me good-bye. "I'll come back whenever you want me."

The days after she left dragged by with nothing but misery for Sam and fear for me. I had felt all along like Sam's jailer, but, after he got back on the transplant list, I began to feel like a grave robber. Every night I would avidly scan the paper for news of bludgeonings, stabbings, and stranglings.

"Here's a good one," I'd say to Sam. "He's down in San Jose and he's still hanging in there, but he's on the critical list. Maybe we'll get him tomorrow." It was gruesome, but it passed the time and gave us something to hope for.

The day Parker came out to California again, Sam went back into the hospital. He had vomited for six straight days, and Dr. Schroeder said over the telephone that the problem was fluid buildup again. Sam would probably have to start being admitted to the hospital two or three times a week to control it.

I had a hard enough time convincing Sam that he should go that morning without giving him that message, and I finally got him admitted through Emergency and bedded down just in time to go up to the airport to get Parker.

Parked in the gun-emplacement parking lot of Emergency, the car flatly refused to go. A sign said emphatically that cars left for longer than one half hour would be towed away. I'd come a long way since Christmas Eve, and the new me did not break down and weep; the new me coped — immodest as it may sound — brilliantly. From Emergency I received unlimited grace as to parking time, and I called the airport from a hospital phone booth, asked to have Parker paged, and left the number of my phone for him to call.

Even Parker, when he finally did call, was impressed. He told me to return to Sam and he would cope with the car, but, an hour later when he still hadn't appeared, I started down the escalator from Sam's floor to reexplore the gun emplacement. Looking down, I saw Parker in the corridor of the floor below, and the new me disintegrated. Nothing and no one had ever looked so wonderful.

"Oh, it's you," I cried with delight, and, forgetting where I was, I tore down the escalator to hug him.

With Parker there everything went right. Sam stopped vomiting. His roommate, recuperating from brain surgery, was wrapped up like an Egyptian mummy and was a grand fellow. We were even visited by Lefty and Mrs. Gomez. Miss Knott brought them to call, and while the former Little League catcher for the Knights of Columbus was impressed, his father was awestruck.

By the next afternoon, after Parker and I had run into Lois Christopherson, I found myself wondering that I had ever despaired. She had only laughed when I confessed my fears to her about Sam's inability to read or write or even follow a television program.

"Of course he can't," she said. "If you had as little blood circulating through your head as he does, you wouldn't be doing half as well. Wait till he gets his heart. The minute he does the whole problem will disappear."

Lois also told us that Sam had just gotten some competition as far as being the second-youngest transplant. "Our youngest one up till now was fifteen years old when we did him two years ago, but he's about to lose his position," she said. "We've got a fourteen-year-old boy here now from Tennessee being evaluated," and Parker and I, walking by the doorway of West I-B where the evaluations were done, saw him.

There was no doubt who he was. He was slowly walking in the hall with a woman who was evidently his mother, and he was thin and frail and grayish blue. "Cardiomyopathy," Parker and I agreed as we went back up to Sam's room, but Sam was not impressed.

"If he's walking in the hall, he's not as sick as I am," he said with un-Christian sourness.

I went home to Portland the night that Sam left the hospital, and I emerged from the plane on the East Coast the next morning feeling strangely confident. I remember saying to Dottie, who met me at the airport, "I know he's going to get his heart while Parker's there. I thought I wanted to be the one who would be with him, but Parker will do it so much better. I'd probably have been so nervous I'd have killed Sam by smashing into something on the way to the hospital. I'll just fly back when the heart comes."

It didn't come the first week I was home. Instead I found an article in the newspaper on heart transplants. "Life Expectancy Increases," said the headline, and I read avidly until I came to the last column. "Six candidates now are waiting at Stanford for a donor heart. All will be dead within three to six months . . . unless a donor heart is found." Sam was one of those candidates.

That ended my optimism with a vengeance, and the telephone calls from California were frustrating. Sam would say "Yeah" or "Okay," but that was about all. Even Alix got distressed.

"He didn't even ask me if I'd lost any weight," she protested sadly one night.

"Count your blessings," I said, but it was disturbing. Parker wasn't much more communicative than Sam. The only time he sounded enthusiastic at all was the night after Sam got a letter from Dr. Bushman.

"Waiting around for things to happen is not always easy," Dr. Bushman had written. ". . . I have seen you in high spirits when I knew you were not feeling well, and the strength of a man is not measured by how much he weighs or how active he can be. It is measured by those other qualities that I have seen in you during our short meetings together."

Thinking about that letter helped, but not enough, because the heart didn't come the next week either. Instead what came was a telephone call from Rozzie with a suggestion from Unkie, Parker's brother. He had spent the night with Parker and Sam in "the plastic," and when he got home to Maine he called Rozzie and told her that Parker's life with Sam had depressed and worried him. "Don't you think it would be a good idea for him to get a nurse or someone who could baby-sit for Sam from time to time so that he could get away from the problem?" he asked.

Rozzie told me she had been very negative about the whole idea. "I told him I'd seen Sam when I was in California, and I didn't think he ought to be left with anyone," she said, "but I told him I'd tell you."

It was a fatal error. I didn't stop to think that Unkie was only trying to help. I didn't stop to think that Sam had probably made an effort while Unkie was visiting and hadn't acted as though he were at death's door. I didn't think about anything. I slammed down the receiver on Rozzie and called California.

"A baby-sitter," I screamed. "For God's sake, Sam is dying, and your brother wants you to get a baby-sitter. What are you going to say to the baby-sitter? 'If Sam dies while I'm out, call me at this restaurant. I'll be back when I've finished my dinner'?"

"Be quiet," Parker said. "There's no baby-sitter. I'll call my brother," and Unkie bravely and foolishly called me that night and apologized.

Poor Unkie, I was dreadful to him, and when Pokie dropped in for his evening visit a half hour later, I was still crying.

He came again the following night, in a highly un-Pokieish manner, with a chrysanthemum plant under his arm. "I thought you needed something to cheer you up,

Mother," he said, and it did for the moment, but the next call from California brought only more despair.

Burpee, the transplant who had not been doing well, had died, and a donor with a matching blood type had been found for the fourteen-year-old boy. He had only had to wait ten days for a heart.

"I keep telling Sam that I'd give him odds an O Negative turns up next time, but it doesn't seem to cheer him up much," Parker said. "He's pretty sunk" — and until Freddie Prinze, the actor, killed himself the next week, the rest of us at home were too.

The entire Maine branch of the family latched on to the idea of Freddie's heart with the tenacity of leaches. Gary Gilmore, the convict who wanted to be executed, hadn't captured our fancies at all, but Freddie Prinze seemed ideally suited for Sam.

"It'll make Sam so unaverage," Ruthie declared. "He'll love it" — and although we never got closer to Freddie Prinze than that, his dying rekindled an enthusiasm in us all that had been absent for days.

On the strength of it, we even got moved into the new addition of the house, but, without Parker to share it with, our new bedroom seemed cold and strange, and the next morning I got up and packed to go back to California even though I wasn't leaving for two more days.

The day before I went back, Alix and Moriah and I went cross-country skiing with Bill and Rozzie and Louise — home from Wyoming for a week — at their winter house.

Throughout our ski, Uncle Bill kept firing questions at me that never seemed to have an answer. "Why didn't they give him Freddie Prinze's heart?" he demanded.

"I don't know," I said, and Rozzie said that Catholics had to go to the grave whole.

"Well, how much longer do you think Sam can last?"
Uncle Bill yelled back at me, as I puffed my way up a
precipitous and rocky incline behind him.

"I don't know," I gasped back. "I just don't know."

By the time we got back to the house, my I-don't-
knows seemed to have taken their toll on Bill. He brought
us a drink in the living room and started pacing his way
from there through the dining room, out into the kitchen,
and back again.

"Somebody's got to do something," he announced, appearing in the room with us and then abruptly heading
back toward the kitchen.

"He's not going to make it if somebody doesn't do something," he said the next time around. On the third trip he
looked at me in total desperation.

"Somebody's got to talk to that fucking God," he said.

The next morning I took Alix intown to a friend's house.
"Good-bye, darling," I said. "I'll be gone when you get
home tonight, but I love you. Let's pray Sammy gets a
heart soon so we can be at home again all at once."

Driving home, feeling a bit weepy, I passed Uncle Bill and
Louise heading for town in their car. Uncle Bill did not
have on his usual Sunday-morning attire. He had on his
Philadelphia hat and coat, and Louise was smiling broadly.

He tooted at me and tipped his hat, and when I got home
I called Rozzie. "Where were he and Louise going at this
hour all dressed up?" I asked.

"He has gone," Rozzie replied with great dignity, "to the
church of his choice to talk to you-know-who."

"Don't worry anymore, Aunt Vic," Uncle Bill directed, as
he drove me to the airport that afternoon. "I've taken care
of the whole matter of Sam's heart at the Unitarian church.
I introduced myself to the minister after the service, ex-

plained that the Episcopal church had done a lousy job on the family funerals, and told him about Sam. He was very impressed. He says he's going to work on the matter of the heart himself, even though I told him I'd handled the whole matter m'sef. Tell Parker and Sam the heart's all taken care of."

I arrived in San Francisco, still shocked but undeniably moved by this new and blasphemous rapport with the Almighty, but Parker didn't even shake his head at my newest "what Uncle Bill has done now."

"Nothing else has worked," he said. "I just hope God heard him, because Sam's got to get a heart pretty soon. The poor kid's running out of gas."

He couldn't have described Sam better. He was lying on the sofa when we got back to the apartment, and he smiled at me and said, "Missed you too," when I told him how awful it had been without him, but the blood cup was full and just the effort of raising his head to kiss me seemed to exhaust him. He was gray and icy cold, lying huddled on his side beneath his blankets, and later, after he'd gone to bed, I clung to Parker. "I wanted him to get it while you were here," I kept saying. "I wanted him to get it so much, and now you have to leave. Oh, I don't want you to go now."

And, being Parker, he said: "I'm not leaving yet. We've got all day tomorrow to catch up."

He was right as always. By the next nightfall we'd walked to the supermarket and told each other everything we'd forgotten to tell each other over the telephone for the past three weeks. I'd told him that it would be much more sensible to be married to someone you hated at moments like this because you'd be so thrilled to have them depart, and he'd told me I'd "never had it so good," but I didn't tell

225

him the decision I'd made the day after Christmas when I thought Sam had died. If I'd told Parker that no one was going to touch Sam until we were both together with him, he would have told me I was wrong and given me good reasons why, and I didn't want him to change my mind.

Sam coughed so badly that night that neither of us slept, and the next morning, which was Groundhog's Day, I told Parker that before he left California he had to go and talk to Dr. Schroeder.

"I want to know where we stand now," I said. "I want to know if he thinks Sam can last to get a heart. If I know where I stand, I can take anything," and to my surprise Parker nodded his agreement and said, "I don't blame you."

He left for the hospital at about nine, and Sam was still in bed when he came back at about quarter past ten. "I found him right off the bat," he announced with satisfaction, "and he says that on balance Sam isn't any worse off now than he's been all along, for what that's worth. Actually he says he's better off than he was when he had the clot because he wasn't even on the list then."

Parker said he'd told Dr. Schroeder that he was leaving that night and that Dr. Schroeder wanted me to be sure to call if I was in any way concerned about Sam, and then he said he guessed he'd walk down to the store and get Sam his newspaper.

It wasn't exactly what I'd hoped Dr. Schroeder would say, but on the other hand I couldn't think of anything else he could have said, so I thanked Parker for going, watched him set off for the store, and sat down at my table, steeled for the next three weeks.

The shuffle to the shower was late that morning. The coughings and gaggings were still coming from the bedroom, and when the phone rang I leapt to answer it before the noise could bother Sam.

"Hello," said a voice. "This is Lois. We think we may have a heart for Sam."

"Oh, my God," I said. "Oh, my God," and I stood there, trying to understand what she was saying so intensely that I never heard Sam come into the room at all.

"What is it?" he said.

And I said, "I think it's your heart," and he grabbed the phone away from me.

"Hi," I heard him say calmly. "What's up?"

Chapter Nine

Before Sam took the telephone away from me, I had heard Lois say something about antibodies and an alternate recipient and two o'clock, but it was all a jumble in my mind. After Sam assumed command, I stood rooted to the spot, hanging on everything he said as if I were being briefed on the Normandy invasion. I should hate to have to hit a beachhead with the information I got from him, however. All he said was "Yeah" or "Okay," and, when the apartment door opened and Parker walked in, Sam was still on the phone and I was in a state of confused shock.

I pointed to my own heart. "It's Lois," I said — I thought quietly — to Parker, and Sam said something that sounded remarkably, although he later denied it, like "Shut up," but the expression on Parker's face made up for any amount of disrespect and for every sad and miserable moment of the past thirteen months. I shall never again say, "How trite," when I read in a book that someone's eyes lit up. Parker's glowed and they sparkled, and, like me, he stood frozen to the spot, listening to Sam.

The commander in chief finally concluded his conversation with a "Thanks, Lois, see ya," and hung up. "It's my heart," he said to us with the utmost composure. "They think they may have one," and he lay down on his sofa.

I was not composed and Parker wasn't either. I kept hugging first Sam and then him, saying, "You can't go home tonight," and Parker kept saying, "I'm not going anywhere, but I don't understand. Schroeder didn't say anything about a heart to me," and Sam grew exasperated with us both.

With our constant interruptions it took him a full ten minutes to make us finally comprehend that a donor was arriving at Stanford sometime during the afternoon, that he, Sam, was to be in the hospital admitting office at two o'clock, and that tests would be run to see if his blood properly matched that of the donor. That was why I had heard Lois talking about antibodies. Enough were evidently present in Sam's blood to cause reasonable doubt that the donor heart would be compatible, and, although if all went well Sam would be the first choice, a backup recipient was coming in too.

It was so marvelous to have something happen and something, at last, to hope for, that neither Sam's irritation with our stupidity nor the prospect that the heart was not a sure thing could dampen Parker's spirits or mine right then. After Sam shuffled off to the shower, Parker called the airline and canceled his flight home.

No sooner had he hung up than the phone rang again. I heard him laugh and say, "Well, you certainly keep a pretty good poker face," and, with surprise, "Really?" and then, "I already have," and finally, "Thanks for calling."

"That was Dr. Schroeder," he said to me. "He didn't know anything about the heart when I saw him. He'd just heard about it and was calling to tell me not to go home tonight."

What we did in the two-and-a-half hours between then and when we went to the hospital I can't remember and I can't even imagine. I know we didn't call anyone at home or at Kent because we wanted to be sure the heart was really Sam's before we did, and I know that Parker and I kept saying that it was a miracle that we were both there together, but the next real picture in my mind is of the three of us sitting in the admissions waiting room at two o'clock — and at two thirty — and at three o'clock — and at three thirty.

We were a credit to our New England upbringing that afternoon; we might to the outward eye have been waiting to have warts removed, and not one of us seemed agitated. Sam and I were on a sofa facing the huge glass entrance doors of the hospital, and Parker sat in a chair adjacent to Sam's with a view of the waiting room itself. The glass doors were automatic, and the long protesting *heeee* as they opened and *haw* as they closed measured out our wait. At first I occupied myself by saying, "There will be five more *heeee*s and four more *haw*s before they call Sam's name," but by two thirty my calculations had proved so incorrect that I abandoned the game and switched to needlepoint. I made so many mistakes so quickly that when a lady came over to admire my handiwork, she departed after one quick glance with a "How unusual," and I put it away.

Parker was silent and inscrutable, and Sam was slumped back on the sofa, paying, as far as I could judge, no attention to anything. I was therefore genuinely startled when he nudged me. "There's the other guy for the heart," he muttered. "I see him at clinic."

I hadn't expected that, and I turned my head and saw, to

our left and just behind us on another sofa, a large young man with very long legs and a dark mustache. He sat very close to a young blond woman, holding her hand, and they were talking quietly. I couldn't hate him. He looked only about Malcolm's age, and if I'd given the matter any thought, I would have realized that of course he had to be admitted too. Right then, however, it seemed macabre to have the two dying contestants for one heart sitting sofa by sofa, practically cheek by jowl. Parker was looking too, and my eyes caught his as I turned back to face the doors.

He just shrugged, though, and then stood up and smiled at me. "Want to share a cup of coffee?" he asked me. "Want some ice, Sammy?" and, when he came back from the cafeteria, he sat in another chair squarely facing the doors.

At three the name Richard Taylor was called. Sam said, "That's him," and I turned again and watched the backup recipient disappear into an office adjoining the waiting room. I looked at Sam and I looked at Parker, but neither lifted so much as an eyebrow. The braying of the doors became intolerable.

We were here first, I thought bitterly to myself. It's not fair; he's going to be admitted ahead of Sam, but I only whispered sourly to Sam, "He doesn't need the heart as much as you do. He isn't even blue."

After that, every minute seemed like another hour. I tried to fold my hands in my lap as an exercise in composure, but they were so ugly to look at and so icy cold that I smoked instead. A tall, tawny, strikingly beautiful girl who could only have been a native of California was standing, with her back to me, in front of the admissions desk, and I pointed her out to Parker. I don't think he even saw her; his lower lip was in and twisting, and the clock said that it was only ten past three.

The backup recipient reappeared and sat down again on his sofa, Sam's name was called, and Parker went into the office.

"Oh, God," I muttered to him when he came back, "if the heart goes to the one who gets admitted first, we're going to lose."

The ridiculous thing is that not one of us can remember who actually did get wheeled off first, or at what time; I can only say that it seemed, at a casual estimate, like three days later. But I shall never forget the trip to the room and the room itself. Both could have been lifted in their entirety from a Frankenstein movie. We were taken to a wing of the third floor, which was not in itself unsettling at all, and we passed by the infant intensive care unit — which was, a bit. The sight of tiny bodies all bandaged and be-tubed always distresses the mother in me, but not until we had progressed beyond the nurses' station and the rows of by-then-familiar Stanford patients' rooms did anything strike me as truly amiss.

When we reached the far end of the hall, familiarity came to a jolting halt. We turned sharply right into a dark, narrow, twisting corridor, and, passing an ominously ill-lit little laboratory and an unstaffed desk on our right, we followed the attendant into another even darker and smaller corridor. At the end of it I could distinguish two open doorways. Sam was wheeled through the first into a room that made any other he had had at Stanford look like the Hall of Mirrors at Versailles. It was minuscule. In it were a bed, a chair, and a basin attached to the wall, and that was it. The foot of the bed prevented the door from closing, and the only daylight in the room came through a deeply recessed vertical glass slit to the right of the bed. The recess was so narrow that my shoulders brushed the sides as I wormed my way to the slit for a view of where we were located; once I got there, what little I could see was splintered and sectioned through a maze of the stucco latticework that surrounds the exterior walls of Stanford Medical Center.

I looked at Parker with horror, but again he only shrugged, and I was left, unnerved, to speculate futilely on the dreadful things they must be going to do to Sam that necessitated putting him in a remote cell, far removed from other patients.

From the doorway I could see a bed turned down in the one adjacent room, and I remember thinking, Oh, God, do you suppose the backup recipient will be in there? — and worse, so much worse that I started to shake: *I'll bet that's where the donor goes!*

Almost immediately, however, technicians started appearing to draw blood from Sam, and I switched from Frankensteinian comparisons to Dracular ones. Vials, test tubes, indeed flagons of blood, it seemed, were drawn and carted away, and until six o'clock none of the three of us had the slightest idea what was going on.

A nurse appeared at that point with a dinner tray for Sam and announced that the donor had arrived at the hospital. By six thirty, when she reappeared to take the tray away untouched, it had become happily apparent that Stanford was not, as I had feared, into horror movies. The empty bed next door had not been gruesomely awaiting either alternate recipient or donor and by then was occupied by a large woman who had had a miscarriage.

I was even able to smile at the nurse when she came back that second time, and Parker asked her if she had any idea when we'd know if Sam could get the heart. She didn't, she said, but she knew the tests took some time, so we waited some more.

Another technician arrived in quest of more blood, and again we waited. The atmosphere in the tiny room was almost unendurably oppressive. Sam didn't speak, and, as the reading light over his bed bothered his eyes, a book was impossible. Parker and I took turns with the chair and turns at going out for a cigarette, and it seemed impossible that the day would ever come to an end.

The nurse went by the door and stuck her head in and Sam said, "I want some ice."

Once a mother, always a mother. " 'I want some ice, *please*,' Sam," I said automatically after the nurse had departed. In retrospect, he was quite justified in giving me a look of pure disgust, but that night I looked right back at him without an ounce of pity. "And there's no need to be rude to me either," I snapped at him and stalked out of the room to have a cigarette.

That was the first argument Sam and I had had in California, and Parker followed me out of the room and, surprisingly, patted my shoulder. "C'mon," he said. "He's upset. It's an awfully rough day for him."

"Of course he is, but there is never an excuse for being rude," I stated implacably.

At about seven thirty, Dr. William Baumgartner, the chief resident for Dr. Shumway's heart transplant team, came into Sam's room in a blue scrub suit, cap, and boots, his surgical mask dangling around his neck. I remember thinking that he looked very young and very tired and that his eyes crinkled in a comforting way at the edges when he smiled at Sam. He stood at the foot of the bed and put a hand on Sam's foot.

"It's a pretty hard day for you, Sam," he said, and his soft voice sounded truly sorry. "Things are looking pretty good, but we have one more test to run. If that checks out all right, you'll be on. We ought to know one way or the other about nine o'clock."

After he left it was as if he had swept the oppressive mood of the room into a bag and taken it away with him, and Sam even shot me a wan smile when he asked the nurse for "more ice, please."

At eight fifteen another scrub-suited form appeared at the foot of Sam's bed. It was the anesthesiologist.

"Does that mean I've got the heart?" Sam asked.

But it didn't. "Not yet, I'm afraid," the anesthesiologist said. "I just thought I'd come and give you a rundown on what we'll be giving you to put you to sleep, if you should get it."

He did, and it was helpful, because his visit consumed another ten or fifteen minutes, but the half hour until the final test was completed dragged away second by second.

"Would you like to call home, Sammy?" Parker asked him, but he shook his head.

"Not now," he said. "Not till we know," and talk subsided again.

We were all three in a partial stupor in the semidarkness of the room, and I never heard Dr. Baumgartner come back into the room, his shoes muffled as they were by surgical boots. I was startled to look over from the basin where I was perched to see him standing at the foot of the bed as if he'd been dropped there from above. The nurse was behind him with a sheaf of papers in her hand.

"How would you like to get a new heart tomorrow morning, partner?" Dr. Baumgartner asked.

He spoke softly, but his voice shattered the silence of the room. Sam shot up out of bed like a balky horse slapped on the rump. He was shaking all over, and he kept lifting first one foot off the floor and then the other, as if he were trying to remember how to jump and couldn't. "Great!" he said over and over, and "Oh, yeah!" and "Thanks."

Dr. Baumgartner looked pleased by Sam's obvious delight. "There are an awful lot of forms here to sign," he said almost apologetically, indicating the sheaf of papers the nurse was carrying, "and I'm sorry, Sam, but we'll have to give you the ATG shots tonight. We want you started on it before the operation. It's a mean way to celebrate getting a heart." He went out the door with a "See you in the morning then, partner."

The nurse started to hand the papers to Parker, but he shook his head and said, "Not me, Sam's eighteen. I think he wants to sign," and she gave them to Sam.

He smiled at her. "Gawd," he said, "I'm the one who's getting the heart, after all," and proceeded to sign himself over to Stanford University and the United States Government as a voluntary participant in all phases of an experimental medical project.

After she departed, the three of us fell upon the telephone and called home. Everyone was asleep, of course, it being midnight on a Wednesday night, but we talked to Ruthie and Malcolm and were halfway through a call to Bill and Rozzie when the nurse reappeared in the doorway, armed with syringes.

"You'll have to have the ATG shots now," she said firmly.

"Can I finish this call?" Sam asked her, but she was relentless.

"No," she said. "Right now," and Sam handed the phone to Parker and swung his legs back up on the bed.

The nurse had four syringes. "Put your legs out straight," she directed, and Sam did.

Parker was still talking to Rozzie as she jabbed the first needle straight down into the top of the upper thigh of

Sam's right leg. It seemed to take an incredibly long time for the syringe to empty, and by the time she drew out the needle Sam's face was contorted and not even grayish blue; it had gone absolutely ashen. Parker was watching as she drove in the second needle. "We'll call back," he said hurriedly, and hung up.

Sam never cried out, but it was terrible to look at his face, and after the final two needles in his left thigh he gasped, "Oh, Christ," and lay back against the pillow with his hands clutching his thighs.

"They say heat helps a little," the nurse said. She produced a large heating pad which she draped over his thighs. "It's supposed to get the stuff moving around." But if it did help, she was right — it was only a little.

I remember feeling very cross with her. She was quite as pregnant as Ruthie, and my heart had gone out to her all the time she had tended Sam, but she had given him the shots so abruptly that he had barely had five minutes of triumph between Dr. Baumgartner's departure and her arrival with the ATG. Plainly, the shots had taken care of triumph with a vengeance, and there would be no more elation that night in the strange little room at the end of the corridors.

There were almost tears from all three of us instead when she came back to the room a little later and gave Sam a note. "Rick Taylor has just gone home," she said. "He asked me to give this to you."

Good Luck, Sam. I'm glad you got the heart. You needed it more than I did.

Rick

It was such a brief message, written on just a scrap of paper — but after Sam read it he said, "Oh, God, what a great guy. I don't think I could have done that," and turned his face into the pillow.

We stayed with him till almost eleven. Parker had had to help him to the bathroom because his legs wouldn't work, but finally he said he thought the pain was a little better, and I kissed him good night. Parker leaned over the bed and held his shoulder. "I'm so proud of you, Sam," he said. "You hung in there all the way. Tomorrow's going to be a great day."

It was easily one o'clock before Parker and I got into bed at the plastic apartment. Each fortified with a large scotch, and showing no respect at all for the hour, we had called Bill and Rozzie back with a long list of people they were to call for us in the morning. At what we've been told was three o'clock Eastern time, we had also called the Perrys at Kent, and Fran answered as coherently as if it were ten o'clock in the morning.

"It's so strange," she said. "I simply couldn't go to bed tonight. I've been sitting here sewing on buttons, as if I were waiting for you to call. We've all been praying for this for so long, and we'll keep right at it, but the school is going to be a zoo when the news gets broken tomorrow."

Parker and I got up at five on Thursday morning, February 3, to go back to the hospital. Sam was to go to the operating room at six thirty, and four hours' sleep was plenty for both of us. "Hurry up," we kept saying to each other as we washed and dressed, and we got to the hospital about six, but the strange little room was empty.

There seemed to be no one in the twisting corridors at the dungeon end of the third floor, so Parker set off to the nurses' station on the main hallway and I waited in the room.

"They couldn't have taken him to the operating room

without our saying good-bye," I kept saying to myself. "They couldn't. He might die and I'd never see him again." I fled the room to find Parker.

As I reached the main hall, I understood why Parker hadn't come back. Sam, in his underdrawers and bare feet, was trying to walk down the hall. He had evidently had a shower because his hair was soaking wet and streamed over his eyes, but his face beneath it was tortured and twisted with pain. He was shaking all over, and his teeth were chattering, and when he took a step his leg jerked straight up from the knee, as if he were a marionette. It threw him off balance, and he didn't seem to go forward at all, but only to stagger from side to side. His right hand kept flailing at the air, brushing away Parker's proffered help.

The progress was interminable, and I stood there, looking at dear Sam's wasted and exhausted body, and knew that if the heart didn't work, and if he should die that day, it was better. Anything was better than his suffering anymore.

When he finally got back to the room, he fell onto the bed, gasping and shivering. "Oh, God, those shots are awful," he moaned. "They hurt so all night, and they made me take a shower, and it was so far away." He was almost sobbing. "I can't walk anymore, Mum."

A nurse and an attendant came with a stretcher then, and Parker and I waited outside the room while they got Sam ready, and when they wheeled him out into the hall, he had a ridiculous pale green shower cap over his wet hair and was still shivering as he lay on the stretcher.

We followed the stretcher down the hallway and took the elevator down one flight with it. The operating-room door was just to the right as we got off the elevator.

"This is it," the attendant said, and I bent over Sam and kissed him.

"I love you," I said.

"Love you both too," he said, and held first my hand for a second and then Parker's.

"Come back with your shield," I called as he went through the door, but I couldn't finish with "or upon it," and Parker called, "Go for it, Sammy," and the operating-room doors closed.

Back in the strange little room collecting his things, one part of me kept saying, I may never see him alive again. His dungarees and sweater, his underdrawers, and the Adidas, bereft of their owner, looked as lost and forlorn as I felt. I could feel the tears coming. Stop it, I ordered myself. Stop it, he's on his way to the top of the glass mountain, and one peril is over: he did live to get a heart.

They had told us that Sam wouldn't possibly get to ICU before one o'clock. Back at the plastic apartment we ate our breakfast, cleaned up, and dressed with all the stately deliberation we could muster, but it was still only ten when we got to the waiting room on the second floor outside the intensive care unit. A long row of chairs faced the reception desk of ICU and the closed double doors that led to the unit itself. Signs on the doors directed that one should introduce oneself to the volunteer at the desk before entering, but having no one yet within the gates, as it were, we didn't.

Instead we sat down. Slipping off my good old traveling off-white coat and putting its arms over the back of my chair, I smoothed my off-white skirt, a companion piece to the now hopelessly uncleanable slacks, and patted the locket around my neck. The night after Mother died, I had come home from Daddy's and, worn out and discouraged, had gone upstairs to kiss Alix good night. She had reached under her pillow and handed me a cheap gold-plated locket I'd bought that fall and had been wearing regularly.

"Look, Mummy," she had said, "it opens." Inside, raggedly cut and placed a bit askew, she had put a snapshot of Mother and, opposite it, a picture of Moriah.

Whatever gold there had been on the locket two years ago had long since worn off, but it was my balm, and I crossed my legs, opened my book, and started to read. Whatever had prompted me to think that a textbook on Russia before the Revolution would make the time while Sam's heart was being cut out pass swiftly, I cannot now conceive. I still know for a fact, however, that Rurik was succeeded in 879 by Oleg, and Oleg by Igor. Their names are permanently engraved upon my mind because I read that sentence — and only that sentence — at least six hundred times while we waited.

At about eleven o'clock, over the top of my book came a little hand smeared with something luridly pink. The hand grabbed my locket.

"Have," a child's voice bleated.

Putting down Rurik, Oleg, and Igor, I saw a little boy of about three.

"Have," he said again, yanking at the locket.

"No," I said, "but I'll open it for you," and I showed him the pictures.

Parker, who does not warm instantly to unknown children and who regularly suggests on airplanes that they go outside and play, shot me a disgusted glance. "You don't have to make friends today," he hissed at me. "Look what he's done to your coat."

I hadn't noticed the child's other hand. It held a large

pink wad of Play-Doh, and while five stained little fingers fondled the locket, five more were massaging the pink into the off-white coat. Looking down at my off-white sweater, I saw that it was rapidly getting pink too.

"Go back to Mummy, dear," I said, trying to detach his fingers one by one without success. Even Parker's "Beat it, kid," which normally sends children flying off in terror, didn't work, but at that the volunteer from the desk appeared and disposed of my little friend.

"Do I have your names?" she asked.

Parker said that we were waiting for Talcott Poole.

"Do you mean you're the parents of the boy who's getting the heart transplant today?" she asked unbelievingly. When we assured her that we were, we had evidently found an admirer.

"How wonderful," she said. "I've been looking at you both and liking you because you seemed so calm. Knowing what you're waiting for makes you even more amazing. You must be from the East. Out here everybody gives way to everything in public. I can't understand it."

She couldn't have given us a kinder compliment at that moment. Inside my head all was angst and primal screams, and Parker admits to having been in equal — if not as tumultuous — distress. It was comforting to be thought controlled.

Our new friend, who told us she was Mrs. Bradford, couldn't do enough to help us. "I'll get a thirty-minute warning, a fifteen-minute one, and a final one five minutes before they bring your son back from the operating room," she said. "I'll let you know every time I hear so you'll know when to look for him. But," she cautioned, "they bring the transplant stretchers back at the most horrendous speed. It's to minimize the chances of contagion going through the hallway, but it's going to look like reckless driving to you. Just close your eyes and don't worry."

She went back to her desk, and I abandoned Rurik and Company altogether. The contemplation of the pink Play-Doh ruins of my chic seemed less taxing to the mind and more absorbing.

Lynn Honma, Sam's ICU nurse, emerged through the double doors of the intensive care unit at about twelve and sat down with us. "The room's all scrubbed," she said. "The hospital had it cleaned last night, but I've been washing every inch of it all over again myself since seven o'clock this morning just so I'll know it's right. We've got everything we're going to need for Sam, and we're all ready, and I'm so excited I can't stand it."

She told us that it would be about an hour after Sam got to his room before we could see him. "We have to get everything running properly and hooked up, and there will be so many people in the room you couldn't get to the bed to see him anyway. I'll come and get you when he's all organized." She bent over and kissed my cheek and vanished back through the double doors, and we sat and waited again.

If he should die, my mind kept saying, remember that you knew this morning that it would be better, but the thought of never seeing Sam again — even sick — was unbearable. The operation is a relatively simple one, I'd tell myself then. That's what everybody's said. But if it's so damn simple, why does it take so long? And I'd look at my watch and then at Parker and say, "Shouldn't he be coming soon?"

At about twenty of one, the phone on Mrs. Bradford's desk rang, and she started smiling at us while she talked. "That's the half-hour warning," she said, after she'd put down the receiver. "Your son is just fine!" and Parker and I abandoned our admired cool and took each other's hand.

Parker was sitting in the last chair in the row on the edge of the hallway through which Sam would come. From that moment on his head was at a permanent ninety-degree angle, as he peered over his shoulder down the hall.

After the final warning, he was on his feet, and finally Sam did come, so fast that the first thing I was aware of was a voice crying, "Get that tube! It's coming out!" At breakneck speed a stretcher came hurtling by to my left. There was a scrub-suited form on either side of it, and two more were galloping along behind it, and, just as someone reached over to adjust something on the body that lay upon it, there was a horrifying crash. The stretcher had barreled into one side of the double doors that Mrs. Bradford was trying to hold open. Parker was at the doorway helping her with the doors and straightening the stretcher while I still sat there. I rushed over just as the stretcher with its escort went flying through the doors and down the hallway inside, but in time to see that it was Sam.

"My God," I said to Parker. "He's got a vacuum-cleaner hose in his mouth. How can he breathe?"

But Parker was so shattered by the collision that all he kept saying was, "If they don't kill him now, they never will."

We were both so absorbed by Sam's abrupt arrival at ICU that we must have forgotten about his doctors. I don't remember giving them the slightest thought, and I was startled when Parker nudged me and indicated two approaching scrub-suited figures. One I recognized from the night before as Dr. Baumgartner; to my surprise, the second turned out to be no other than Dr. Shumway himself.

"I don't see how he made it," he said, shaking his head. "I just don't see what kept him alive. The walls of the heart were as thin as paper, and the whole thing was dead tissue — all fibrous and spotted just like a leopard hide. We've sent it down to pathology, but I know there wasn't enough live tissue for us to ever find out what caused his cardiomyopathy."

And Dr. Baumgartner said, "The heart just fell apart when we touched it."

It was even harder to wait after that. Parker says we called home from the ICU waiting room, but I don't remember it. I can only remember Lynn running toward us through the inner doors of ICU, her almond-shaped eyes dancing with delight, crying: "Come on! Come on! He's all ready for you."

We almost ran behind her, back through the doors, and were nearly at the end of the long inner corridor when she stopped at a closed door on the left.

"Here we are," she said. "I'll help you dress."

A cart with two shelves on it stood to the right of the door, piled high with shapeless blue-wrapped packages. Lynn was laughing and talking both at once as she handed them to us and tried to get us into them. The blue paper boots we put on over our shoes went on easily, and the bonnet and the mask. I even managed somehow to get into the gown, which tied in two places in the back, but my hands were so clammy and awkward I ripped the first plastic glove I tried to get on, and I remember thinking, Oh, we'll never get to see him, as I fumbled on the cart for another pair.

Lynn was standing on her tiptoes, trying to wedge Parker into a gown whose duplicate on her was all-encompassing, crying "He's too big!" and when we finally were all covered, I remember thinking, We'll scare him to death dressed like this.

But once we'd followed Lynn into the room, how we looked wasn't of any consequence. Another nurse, almost as tiny as Lynn, was bending over the bed, and when she turned to smile at us, I saw Sam — the Sam I'd known before this awful year. He was sleeping peacefully, and there wasn't a vestige of the dying boy I'd seen at six thirty that morning. The slew of tubes and the huge hose taped in his mouth which connected him to the respirator were the only reminders that in the morning he had truly looked more dead than alive. His cheeks were pink, and he was pink and white all over, and he was handsome, even with his mouth so oddly shaped to accommodate the hose. He hadn't been, before. I guess it's only in books and movies that somebody who's dying is handsome.

"Oh, Lynn," I said, "can I feel his feet?" and when she nodded I picked my way through tanks and machines and wires to stand at the foot of the bed, and they were warm! They were pink too, and I kissed his toes through my mask and just stood there patting them.

He's Thursday's child now, I kept thinking. Thursday's child has far to go.

I could have stayed there forever looking at him. For his part, Parker couldn't tear his eyes away from the heart monitor over the bed. "My God," he'd exclaim, "it makes me feel like a million dollars to see that thing ticking away like that."

When Dr. Baumgartner came into the room a few hours later, at about six, he just shook his head at the two of us still standing there. "Sam's going to be asleep for a long time yet," he said. "Why don't you go home and get some rest yourselves? He'll want you in the morning."

He told us that Sam would be extubated by then, which I remember Lynn telling me meant that the hose would be taken out of his mouth and the tubes pulled out of his chest. She had said that pulling the chest tubes could be awfully painful, but as Dr. Baumgartner left the room, he smiled at us and said, "Sam may still be so groggy when we pull them, he won't mind it too much."

Chest tubes seemed a small matter, and, with one last check of his toes by me and of his monitor by Parker, we left the room, knowing that we had seen a miracle. There is simply no other way to describe it; it was, it *was* a miracle.

When Parker and I got back to the apartment that night, there was a telegram for Sam in our mailbox. It said: I TOLD YOUR UNCLE I WOULD GIVE HIM ANYTHING HE WANTED IF HE WOULD LOWER HIS VOICE. I NEVER HEARD SUCH DREADFUL LANGUAGE. It was signed, THE LORD.

Chapter Ten   At Kent School the bells of St. Joseph's Chapel rang for Sam's new heart. In Dedham, Massachusetts, Ruthie's mother wrote on a big red cardboard heart: *Sam Poole — No. 1 Heart Throb — Valentine's Day is February third forevermore!* And in Portland the minister at the church of Uncle Billy's choice was astounded to hear that Unitarians had such close rapport with the Lord.

At the Cape, Ruthie wrote: "What a day! The most exciting, most meaningful, most stupendous, most nerve-racking, most telephoned about, most toasted, most prayed about, most relieving, relaxing, exhausting day in the world!" and Freddie Gemmer's father covered an entire sheet of paper with one word — HOORAY!

In the plastic apartment, however, Parker and I wandered about in a daze. Having never witnessed a miracle before, we relived every minute of ours with awe, and it took Sam himself to shatter the aura of sanctity that surrounded him.

"Heart Transplant One-twenty wants his Adidas," Lynn said when she called us the next morning.

248

"He wants what?" I gasped. "Those sneakers must be crawling with germs. I thought he had to be kept sterile."

"Oh, he does," Lynn said, "but after all, he'll be having books and stuff in his room. He'd go stir crazy if he didn't. It's the germs people carry we really worry about. Just scrub them up inside and out as carefully as you can."

"What on earth does he want those rotten shoes for?" I kept asking Parker, but there's nothing like cleaning old sneakers to start putting things back into perspective, and once we'd seen Sam's door after we got to ICU, we were both securely tied back to earth again.

In my excitement to see him the day before, I hadn't noticed the door. Just as if it were a speakeasy, there was a little wooden panel about two-thirds of the way up. Lynn had decorated the rest as if it opened onto the first day of kindergarten. A piece of yellow cardboard informed us in bright red and importantly flourishing letters that this was SAM'S ROOM. Beneath that was another piece of paper with a big red heart on the left and the word TRANSPLANT after it. BE THE ENVY OF ALL YOUR FRIENDS, the paper advised, directing attention to a drawing of a ludicrously dressed human form. To ENTER THIS ROOM YOU MUST WEAR: *#1 Boots, #2 Hat, #3 Mask, #4 Gown (preferably wrinkled, some wit had penciled in), and #5 Gloves.* Arrows went from the words to the picture so there would be no doubt as to where on the anatomy the items went, and Lynn had drawn flowers all over the gown and colored the boots and the mask red.

It was nice to know that ICU wasn't going to be intimidating, but without Lynn to help us, dressing was even more frustrating than it had been the day before. What I wanted to do was rush into the room and see Sam, but what we had to do — with many references to the chart for sequence —

was sort out the packages on the cart. I did notice, as I hadn't the day before, that the hard blue plastic mask smelled atrocious and that the sea-foam green of the bonnet was not Parker's color, but mostly I remember thinking, Oh, God, it's taking us longer to get dressed than we're allowed in the room. I had seen fierce signs that said ICU visiting time was fifteen minutes.

When we finally were ready, Parker knocked very softly. "He might be asleep," he whispered. Neither of us was prepared for the noise when Lynn opened the door. It was a voice we hadn't heard for more than a year. It was loud, and it was determined, and it was protesting.

"Food! I need food! That wasn't a meal, Lynn. I'm a growing boy," it said, and there, less than twenty-four hours after his operation, sitting up in bed, was Sam. In front of him was a tray without a crumb left on it.

He was grinning from ear to ear, his eyes were wide open, and his hair, which looked as if it had been brushed for the first time in ages, gleamed gold in the sun that poured through the wide window next to his bed. The lank dirty-blond straggles I remembered from the morning before seemed to have vanished overnight, and the hand that pointed with dismay to the empty tray was blue-nailed no longer.

"Hi, Mum. Hi, Dad. Isn't it great?" he said. I simply couldn't believe him. Parker had groaned for three days after his hernia operation.

"Oh, Sam, you're beautiful!" I cried, and rushed over to the bed.

When I got there I didn't dare hug him. The heart-lung machine was gone, but there was so much attached to him that I only bent over and gingerly gave him a peck on the cheek through my blue mask and tore to the end of the bed to squeeze his feet and pat his toes.

"Mu-um," he deplored.

"I don't care. I'm going to pat them every day; I just love them," I said firmly. "I've earned patting them," and then, looking at him, I really took in his incision for the first time. A scar to me is my appendix scar, wide, bluish purple all over, sunken in the middle and bulging on both sides — in short, an eyesore. Sam's was obviously going to be an artistic conversation piece in time. It was tidy and much thinner than I had expected. There were no outer stitches at all, but it did stretch from his neck to just above his waist, and there was no denying that it was intimidating.

"Oh, Sam," I said, "you look so marvelous, I forgot. Does it hurt?"

To my complete surprise he said, absolutely emphatically, "Not a bit!" He sat up even straighter in bed without a twinge, took a long deep breath, held it for a second, and, with a look of pure joy, let it out again. "See?" he said triumphantly, "I can breathe again, and it doesn't even hurt."

Tears were stinging my eyes, and some must have been stinging Parker's too, because I heard a distinct sniff and he cleared his throat before he said, "Gosh, Sammy, Dr. Baumgartner even took a detour around your birthmark. That's pretty tricky, huh?"

I remember thinking then, Oh, Lord, we mustn't tire him out; our fifteen minutes must be up. But Sam's face fell when I suggested to Parker that we ought to leave.

"But you just got here," he protested with such genuine dismay that Lynn started to laugh.

"Do you want them to stay, Sam?" she asked, and when he said, "God, they haven't seen half of me yet," she told us something we'd never heard before. At Stanford, visiting rules never apply to heart transplants. *They* make the decisions about who visits them and for how long.

"You can stay all night, if Sam wants you to," Lynn said, still laughing, and we settled back to marvel some more.

There were so many things to wonder at. Gone from the screen of the heart monitor was the erratic pattern of his old heart, and beautifully regular beeps now came as steadily as the ticks of a clock. Beneath the two rubber cups on his chest which connected him to the monitor, Lynn told us, there were two blue tattoos.

"He'll be having electrocardiograms all the time and forever," she explained. "With the tattoos there they'll always put the wires on the same spot, and there'll be no variance in the readings from positioning."

And the bandage at the bottom of the incision? That was where his chest tubes had been pulled out.

"You wouldn't believe Sam," she said. "He must be a stoic or else he doesn't have any feeling. He never even winced when the tubes came out, and usually that's the worst part of the whole operation. Maybe he's just dumb." She giggled, patting his shoulder in the fondest way after she had removed a bandage from the left side of his neck.

A needle with a short, hard, white plastic tube attached was protruding from the base of Sam's neck under the bandage. The hard tube — or shunt, as Lynn called it — had two holes at the top to accommodate soft plastic tubing, which in turn was attached to bottles hanging on the IV pole next to the bed. There was a third hole in the shunt, and she bent over Sam and emptied a syringe into it.

"The shunt's great," she said. "Sam would be a pincushion if we had to give him his meds with separate needles every time," and when she listed the number of drugs he was receiving through it, I wholeheartedly agreed with her. Only a blood tranfusion, dripping down from another IV pole, was being given by independent needle in his right arm.

The shunt was conveying massive amounts of diuretics, steroids, and God knows what all from the hanging bottles into Sam's bloodstream now, but Lynn explained that either most of those drugs would be discontinued in time or Sam would start taking their oral equivalents. She walked over to a huge chart tacked on the bulletin board on the wall facing Sam.

"I've been very busy with my red Magic Marker, as you can see," she said, "but there are so many drugs Sam has to cope with, I thought this might help. These are the meds he's taking orally now, and all but one of them he'll probably be taking for the rest of his life. Taking medicines five times a day gets confusing, and what Sam has got to start learning right away is how, when, and in what order he takes them. He's got to know just what they're doing to him. By the time he leaves ICU, he'll know his medications as well as, if not better than, his doctors."

A less likely looking professor than Lynn there never was. Little wisps of dark wavy hair had escaped from beneath her bonnet, and, with her gown dragging on the floor and the huge blue paper booties protruding from beneath it, she looked — as I told her — more like Minnie Mouse.

The chart was divided into three sections. On the left, each drug was listed; in the middle, under a column headed ACTIONS, was the purpose of each; and on the right, the drug's side effects. There were a lot of side effects listed for the first two drugs, prednisone and Imuran. Both were immunosuppressants, and both would be taken in pill form.

"I know Lois told you in December about the chipmunk

cheeks and the potbelly that go along with taking pred- nisone," Lynn said, "and you've probably all seen people who are taking it in some form or other. Unfortunately there's not much you can do about the cheeks, but the pot- belly's another matter. If I know you, Sam, you're going to be too vain to let that sneak up on you, so if you exercise enough *and* watch what you eat, you can keep it under con- trol. It's not going to be easy, though, because prednisone makes you ravenously hungry all the time, and just to make matters worse it causes stomach irritation too."

That wasn't all prednisone did. It caused wide stretch marks to appear like scars on the skin and, even worse, it could trigger wild mood swings.

"Sam could be as happy as a clam one morning," Lynn explained, "and by afternoon feel as if he'd lost his last friend. It varies from patient to patient, but now, while he's taking such massive doses, he's sure to have some ups and downs. That's one reason why there is always a nurse in the room twenty-four hours a day. The swings can be frightening for both the transplant and his family."

Imuran, the other immunosuppressant, posed problems for the future — bone marrow depression and a decrease in white blood cells. It sounded frightening, but I tried not to think of future problems.

Don't trouble trouble, I scolded myself. Happily there were no side effects listed for the third drug, Persantine. Lynn said it kept platelets from sticking and prevented clot formation in the blood. It was taken in pill form too.

The next drug on the chart, named with a groan from Lynn, was ATG. "That's the shots, you know, Sam. It's real name is anti-thymocite globulin, and even though it hurts so dreadfully when it's injected, it's really the key to Stan- ford's success with heart transplanting. Everybody calls it

Dr. Shumway's secret weapon because it suppresses antibodies and prevents rejection better than anything else, but along with the pain it sometimes causes fever. At least, though," she said with a wry smile, "there's no ATG in Maine, so unless you start rejecting badly at home and have to come back to Stanford, you'll be finished with it when you leave California, if that's any comfort."

There were no side effects listed for the fifth, sixth, or seventh drugs. Titralac was a pill that counteracted the stomach irritation caused by prednisone, and Mycostatin was a lozenge that prevented oral yeast infections. After that came Stanford mouthwash, which didn't sound like a drug at all, and Lynn laughed for the first time since she'd started to go over the chart. She went to a little table near the entrance of the room where innumerable bottles and jars were stacked and picked up a bottle filled with the vilest-looking liquid I'd ever seen. It wasn't mint green; it wasn't lime green; it was a green that could only be associated with leprechauns, and it looked thick and syrupy.

"Stanford's very proud of it," Lynn said. "It's their own concoction, and it's supposed to work miracles on germs, but the color? My God!"

The next drug, Coumadin, wasn't amusing at all. It was an anticoagulant, or blood thinner, and I already knew firsthand about its side effects. It was Coumadin that had sent Sam and me rushing to the emergency room on New Year's morning a month before. It caused bleeding from the stomach and lungs as well as excessive bruising and bleeding from cuts.

"You've got to be awfully careful from now on about not bumping into things, Sam," Lynn said. "That's why all contact sports are off the list for transplants. What amounts to a little bump for other people could turn into a hemorrhage for you. You'll even have to be terribly careful when you shave."

There came an almost forgotten noise from the bed, sounding somewhere between a sneer and a guffaw. I hadn't heard it for so long it took me a second to remember that it was Sam's chortle.

"I'll grow a beard," he gloated, "and next year at Kent when Mr. Perry tells me to shave it off, I'll tell him if I do I'll bleed to death. I'll get to be the first kid at Kent with a beard." Only when Lynn ordered him to pay attention did he stop stroking his bare chin as if he already had a foot-long growth on it.

Lasix was the next-to-the-last drug on the chart and was a diuretic, or water pill. The only bad thing it seemed to cause was potassium loss. "You'll take powdered potassium three times a day to replace it, Sam," Lynn said and then pointed to the last drug, which after the others didn't seem exciting at all. It was Colace, a pill that softened stools and only caused diarrhea.

"Oh, Lord, Lynn," I said, "how many pills or powders or what-all will he have to take every day?"

To someone who can barely choke down an aspirin, her answer was appalling. "He'll probably end up taking about fifty or so," she said. "It varies, because sometimes one drug is cut down and another one is increased, and in time other drugs may be added to the list. I know it sounds wild, and it's going to take a long time for Sam to learn them all, but it's his responsibility. He can't leave ICU until he can take them alone. When he does go he's got to remember that, miserable side effects and all, they're the only way he's going to stay alive. If he doesn't take them —"

She didn't say anything more, but her usually twinkling brown eyes, framed as they were by the mask and the bonnet, were so deadly serious she didn't have to. I turned my head and tried to look at the chart objectively, but the words *bone marrow depression* and *bleeding from stomach, lungs* were all I could see.

I was sitting on the window ledge. I wanted to jump up and scream, "It's not fair. He's only eighteen," but instead I just swallowed hard. You knew it, I thought. All along you knew things could never go back to where they were before he got sick. He's alive! If the price he has to pay for being alive is all those damned drugs tearing his insides to pieces, at least he's alive. But the list of medicines was long and frightening. I tore my eyes away from it to see that Sam, completely unperturbed, was peering down at his chest.

"Hey, Lynn," he said, "I've got wires coming out of my insides. What are those for?"

I hadn't noticed them before either, but two wires were certainly protruding from two holes below and to the right of his incision. He was electrified as authentically as if he were a Christmas tree. The two wires were attached to a flat electric plug, which in turn was attached to another wire. I followed that one up to the top of the IV pole, from which hung a gray box about the size of a medium-sized transistor radio.

"Oh, that's your pacemaker," Lynn said. "That's so your heart will beat consistently, at an even rate. There's a good chance you won't need it after you've had the heart awhile, but right now it's a good precaution."

"Of course I won't need it," Sam said with the utmost authority. "My new heart likes me; I can feel it. Boy, am I glad I don't ever have to know where it came from or whose it was. I don't ever want to know. It's my heart now, and nobody's going to take it away from me."

I remember thinking, What a funny thing to say, but I didn't dare ask him why he felt that way, and instead to change the subject I held up the sneakers, which were next to me on the window ledge.

"Can I ask just one question?" I said. "With all that stuff attached to you, Sam, what on earth do you want these for?" The minute I looked at his face I wished I hadn't asked.

"I'm going to hug them," he said with disgust. "I'm gonna stick my thumb in my mouth and hug them. Gawd, Mum, whadda ya think I want them for? Lynn says I can go to the can after this transfusion is done but not in bare feet. I might catch cold. Gawd, you women! You'd keep me in bed for the rest of my life."

"Sam Poole, you're *horrible*," Lynn said. "Just for that I ought to tie you to the bed," but after the transfusion was finished, she detached him from the heart monitor, and he swung his legs effortlessly over the side of the bed and shoved his feet into the sneakers.

He'd lost 51 pounds while he was sick. The last day at clinic he'd weighed 126 pounds, and his arms were so thin I could have circled them with my hand. Standing there towering over Lynn, with nothing on but the sneakers and hospital-pajama bottoms, he looked like a battered old scarecrow. But without even leaning on her he smiled and walked off quickly toward the bathroom as Lynn scurried beside him guiding the IV pole. Parker and I could only watch in amazement. He was still smiling when he got back into bed, but for him it was evidently peeing (in the Stanford vernacular), not walking, that was his triumph.

"I'm my own man again," he crowed. "I hate those damned catheters."

Still amazed, I said accusingly, "You're showing off,

Sam. It's got to hurt to walk. You can't have your chest split in two and not have it hurt. It does hurt him, doesn't it, Lynn?"

"No," she said, "not Sam. I guess he is dumb."

"Mum, nothing could ever hurt like it did before," Sam said. "They could have carved me up the back and down both sides too, and it wouldn't hurt the way just breathing did. I guess Randy felt the same way too. Look," and he handed us a note from the fourteen-year-old transplant.

Hi, Sam,

Hope you're feeling as well as I did after I got my chest tubes out. I slept through mine. Keep that monitor ticking and those legs a pumping.

Randy

"What a pair those two are," Lynn said, shaking her head. "They act as if all they had were colds in the head."

Sam generously conceded that Randy sounded okay. "I called him on the phone and told him so," he said. "I even told him I didn't hold it against him that he only had to wait ten days for a heart."

I couldn't believe anything by the time we went home for supper. We'd spent practically the whole day in Sam's room, and he was looking just as perky as he had in the morning. He'd even told us to be sure to eat quickly so we'd be back in his room in time for his shots. I took all the memories of his first healthy day to bed with me that night. Even the misery on his face as the ATG shots were given that evening and the cautions of Lynn's chart — *bleeding from stomach, lungs* and *bone marrow depression* — were no match for his first phone call home at noon, designed to coincide with Alix's return from school.

"Hi, Al. Didn't get rid of me, did ya? Hey, Al, I watched the whole thing. They asked me if I wanted any anesthesia and I said no, and it was just great. I saw all the knives and all the blood, and when you have your tonsils out I'm gonna tell the doctor you don't wanna be put to sleep either."

Armed with that I snuggled down under the dreadful red fuzzy blanket as if it were ermine and slept along with Parker for nine straight hours.

It didn't take us any time at all to get used to the long rows of pill cups lined up on the tabletop swung over Sam's lap in bed.

"What's that?" Lynn would ask, pointing to four little round red pills.

"Prednisone?" Sam would ask hopefully.

"No, Sam. That's Persantine. What does it do to you?" And, after he'd answered, she'd ask, "What's that?" pointing to another.

Once Parker corrected him, and Sam snapped back, "You take your pills, Dad, I'll take mine," and neither of us ever dared make a comment again. After we met Judy, who came on duty with Sam in the afternoons after Lynn's shift was over, however, we all snickered when the medicine lesson got to Mycostatin.

Judy had thick, jet-black braids that kept slipping out from her bonnet; high cheekbones; and dark, inscrutable eyes. She had seemed a very subdued replacement for Lynn, who filled the room with chatter and teasings, and for the first hour she was with Sam she said very little. When it came time for his medicines, she stood impassively watching Sam suck his Mycostatin lozenge.

260

"Did Lynn tell you what Mycostatin is, Sam?" she asked solemnly.

All three of us shook our heads.

It was the most startling transformation. The eyes crinkled wickedly, and from behind the mask came a wonderfully silly giggle. "It's a suppository for women with VD," she said, as the patient stopped sucking with an expression of pure horror on his face.

Mycostatin taken care of, the eyes uncrinkled, solemnity returned, and, in answer to a question of Parker's about ATG, she started to explain with complete sobriety what it was and where it came from — the thymus gland.

Everyone is born with a thymus gland, she told us. It gives immunity during the prenatal period, but apparently its function ceases after birth, and it gradually dissolves. When they do chest surgery on infants, the gland gets in the way and is removed, and at some point Dr. Shumway thought of putting it and its immune properties to work for his transplants.

"What makes the ATG hurt so," Judy said, "is that it's almost pure protein. They're always experimenting to try to make the serum less painful, but they haven't come up with anything yet."

I was listening so intently that I didn't see the eyes crinkle again. "They used to use somebody's old horse to make the serum," Judy said. "They'd scramble up the baby thymus glands and inject them into the horse, but one night some drunk ran over it while its blood was right in the middle of making a batch. They say Dr. Shumway was fit to be tied. There he was with all his transplants and no ATG. They've had to use rabbits since then." The eyes uncrinkled. "Somehow rabbits aren't the same," she said wistfully. "I always liked the idea of the old horse, munching away in his pasture, keeping all the transplants going."

It was that way with everything Judy told us. There was always something at the end that took the formidable away from heart transplanting and made it almost cozy. It was interesting, for example, to know that if Sam walked right off the street into a doctor's office, the doctor would know just by looking at his EKG tape that he was a heart transplant.

"No one else has two starters," she explained. "When a transplant is done, the starting mechanism for the old heart isn't removed, and the donor's starter comes along with the new heart. Look," she said, and pulling off a piece of the tape that spewed out of Sam's heart monitor, she marked with a blue arrow the little bump on the heartbeat line where Sam's old heart started and with a red one the bump where the donor's starter kicked in.

"God, that's fascinating," I said, but to this day I don't understand if having two starters is a good thing or a bad thing.

One thing she told us I knew was going to be bad. Parker was going home to Maine that night because Sam was doing so well there was no excuse for both of us to hover around him, and just before we left his room to go to the airport, Sam said, "I wish I could drive you up, Dad. Just think, in a couple of months I'll be able to."

"He may not want you to drive him anywhere, Sam," Judy said. "When they took out your old heart, they severed the nerve that goes to your brain, and they can't reattach the donor's to yours. Do you know that it will take you a good two or three minutes to pump up enough adrenaline to be able to react the way people do when they're in panic?"

262

"So what's wrong with that? Why's that so bad?" Sam asked defensively. "I can't stand people screaming around all over the place."

The eyes crinkled; the giggle began. "It isn't bad for you, Sam," she said, "but it's pretty awful for the people driving with you. If you were about to smash into something going eighty miles an hour, it wouldn't bother you a bit."

I mulled that over all the way up the freeway. "I can hardly wait to have him drive me somewhere," I said gloomily.

Parker refused to be ruffled. "Think how Sam will love it," he said. "He always likes to play things cool."

He was equally unruffled at being left off at the curb outside the terminal three hours early for the red-eye special, which didn't leave till ten. ATG shots were given at eight thirty, and it was already indelibly imprinted on our minds that family support above all meant being with Sam before, during, and for a good two hours after the fateful twelve cc's were injected. By comparison, Parker said, a three-hour wait for a plane was peanuts.

The shots had been the hardest thing to get used to. I had asked Judy why they had to be given at night. "Sam dreads them all afternoon," I'd said, but her answer had been completely reasonable.

"If he had them in the morning he'd dread them all night," she said, "and his legs would be so sore he'd never want to get out of bed." It was no comfort to hear that with each successive night the shots would be worse, as the ATG broke down Sam's leg muscles.

"Don't you worry about Sammy," Parker said as he leaned through the car window to kiss me good-bye. "He got through the wait; he'll get through the shots. That kid's awful tough," and, even though anguish had to be Sam's

263

evensong, I was able to say, "Good-bye, I love you," with a smile.

For anybody's information, tending a heart transplant is a full-time occupation, and three days passed before I even realized that for the first time in my forty-nine years I was living alone and could take time to wonder if I was doing it properly. The plastic apartment was not in a savory neighborhood — only two blocks away was the street ominously referred to as Whiskey Gulch — and its garage was ill lit and subterranean. A precipitous hill led you off Woodland Avenue down into open stalls from which, having left the car, you progressed not back uphill to the street, but through a dark passageway to a locked door that led up to the apartments. I didn't get home from the day's last visit to the hospital until well after ten thirty at night, and it crossed my mind that no one would know if I never did. Visions of a dead me, sprawled undiscovered on the concrete of the garage, prompted an inspired solution. I sang in my dreadful monotone at the top of my lungs, hoping that at least someone other than a potential assailant would hear me. The pussycat who lived on the floor below us did. From the first note he would start to howl from his balcony, and having thus acquired a watchcat, I forgot about being nervous.

I didn't even have time for my vices. I left Sam's room in the evening at six, and, as it took a good ten minutes to get to the plastic, I had barely time for one drink while I heated my stove-top dinner. Having gobbled it down, I leapt into the car to be back in his room by seven. When I got home again at almost eleven, I would take a shower and curl up under the red fuzzy blanket with my book and a second drink. At least that's what I did at the beginning, but I never could stay awake to drink it. After several mornings of waking up to the dreadful stench of undrunk scotch, I abandoned that habit; and with no smoking in Sam's room, I barely had time for my daily quota of nicotine. I felt very virtuous.

I reported back to the hospital for duty at ten o'clock in the morning, bearing, as my entry ticket to Sam's room, ten sugar-free homemade popsicles; Sam's appetite, the first evident side effect of prednisone, had become insatiable. The first word we'd heard him say after his operation had been "food," and it had rapidly reached a crescendo.

"Look at me," he would bleat to anyone who would listen to him. "Skin and bones, that's all that's left! I oughta weigh a hundred and seventy-five pounds, for God's sake."

For several days Lynn kept the bleats under control by appealing to his vanity. "Sam, you're not getting any exercise. You'll get fat. I thought I saw a little potbelly this morning," and he would suck in his breath and nervously pat his stomach and meekly suggest that "one little cup custard couldn't be that fattening."

Eventually, however, the bleats became wails, and she sent for the dietitian. The dietitian was unmoved.

"You're eating over thirty-five hundred calories a day, Sam," she said. "That's more than you need by a long shot, and, no, you can't eat popsicles in between meals to keep you full. They have sugar in them. Remember, if you're planning to stay alive, it's no cholesterol, no salt, and no sugar."

But even that warning couldn't quell his complaints. His conversational gamut went only from "I'm hungry" to "Isn't it almost time to eat?" until Dottie heard his laments over the phone. She suggested freezing orange juice in a paper cup with a plastic spoon in the middle. "Don't you remember, Sam?" she said. "That's what I always did at the cottage in the summer when you guys were little." Stanford's nutrition department thought it was a great idea. After that, making and meting out Dottie's popsicles to Sam to conform with his allowed daily caloric and liquid intake became a central theme to our days.

"You get all your meds straight tonight, Sam, and I'll let you have one more," Lynn would say.

And "Oh, my God!" I'd shriek, leaping out of bed at three in the morning. "I forgot to put the popsicles in the freezer!" Suicide, I knew, would be a cheerful alternative to arriving popsicleless at 10 A.M. at Sam's door.

Hunger, the first side effect of prednisone, was rapidly followed by a second, mood swings, but with Sam the swing only went in one direction — up. He got cheerier and cheerier every day, which no one could complain about. One afternoon, however, after he had ravenously but quite sanely devoured his lunch and was napping peacefully, the telephone rang. It was Freddie Gemmer. I shook Sam and handed him the receiver. He didn't make any sense at all, and after five minutes of incoherent mumbles, it became apparent that he was not sleepy but drunk.

He giggled, he slurred his words, and he finally said, "Geez, Fred, I dunno where I am. Where the hell are you? Waita min't — here's my mother. She knows where I am," and, shaking his head, he handed me the phone and with a "Too much f'r me" he lay down.

"Is he all right, Mrs. Poole?" I heard Freddie's voice asking nervously.

"I guess so," I said, just as nervously. "I think he's gotten drunk without you, Fred. I'll have him call you tomorrow." But when I got back to the hospital after supper, I began to wonder if Sam would be sober even by then. He was still giggling helplessly, and Judy was staring at him.

"He's gone crazy," she said. "The prednisone's gotten to him. He *drank* his Stanford mouthwash. He sat right there in bed and drank it." And she held up an empty paper cup, still rimmed with the atrocious-looking green stuff, as testimony.

"Did tashte pretty awful, Judy," Sam finally got out when he stopped laughing. "Maybe m'shtill drunkenuf notta feela shots." And although that was too much to hope for, by the time I went home at eleven, he was sound asleep, with a smile on his face.

"The patient is feeling no pain," Judy whispered, as I bent over to kiss him good night.

Although Sam never again got drunk on prednisone, most of the time he was as silly as if he were. Only as shot time approached did he retreat into silence, and then with good reason, but the rest of the day he was entirely himself.

"He is a 'wonder of wonders, miracle of miracles,' " I wrote to Tina in England, interspersing musical notes at random above and below the words, "and such a Sam again. He talks all day, he smiles, he gives the average-Joe pitch, he is, to quote your papa, 'something else!' "

Somewhere along the line, though, it began to dawn on me that Sam was a lot more than just his old self. It began with the nurses. When we had been told that a nurse would be on duty with Sam twenty-four hours a day, we had been told the truth; Lynn or Judy couldn't even leave the room for a ten-minute break without being relieved by another properly garbed nurse, and Sam greeted each unrecognizable substitute with unfailing good cheer.

"I never have any trouble getting someone to sign up for you, Sam," Lynn told him one day. "All the nurses say they

267

come in here for a rest." I was sitting reading on the window ledge, and she turned to me and said, "You know, it's true, Mrs. Poole. No one can believe Sam. He even smiles and says thank you for the ATG shots."

"Of course he does," I said. "He has a remarkable mother who brung him up good," but Sam didn't even take time to sneer at me.

"Hell, Lynn," he said. "Why take my troubles out on everybody else? It's not their fault I got sick. The greatest gift for me is just being here. I oughta make it easy for people. All along when I was sick, I'd just lie there and tell myself that I'd make myself live till they got a heart for me because I wanted one so bad. God, I can't screw up now and make it rotten for the people who are trying to help me do it. I gotta do it right."

It wasn't just compassion for the people who helped him either. He didn't even demand his popsicle when I walked into the room one morning.

"Geez, Mum," he said, "did you know Randy's older brother died two years ago of cardiomyopathy? Randy told me over the phone this morning. The doctors said his brother had acid indigestion, just like me, and, by the time they discovered it wasn't, it was too late. He just died. God, what a bad deal."

He was quiet for a minute, and then he said, "Mum, you know you and Dad oughta have Al checked out. She oughta have a chest X-ray. Promise me you'll do it when you go home."

I promised, and as every day went by I realized more and more that, even though he couldn't leave his room and had never met any of his fellow transplants, their problems had become his problems too. He sweated out the results of each one's biopsy, Stanford's method of detecting rejection, as if it were his own, and he hadn't even had his heart long enough to need a biopsy or to reject. His concern was contagious, and as I found myself worrying too, I began to realize that recipients and their families became members of the Stanford transplant team quite as thoroughly — if not as effectively — as the doctors and nurses themselves. It was surprising to find myself rooting for teammates for the first time in my life.

In truth, it wasn't a large team. There were only two other transplants in ICU then, interspersed along the hall among the other intensive care patients. Randy's room was down near the doors that led to the waiting room, and at the other end of the hall, in the room next to Sam, was a Mr. Terrence, whom everyone referred to as Terry and who was, everyone admitted, "awfully old for a transplant." Terry had gotten the heart on January 7 that I'd wrongly prophesied would be Sam's.

Across the hall in the self-care section, separated from ICU proper by nurses' stations, diet kitchens, and conference rooms, was a third transplant — Cobbie, the one with a penchant for beer. Lynn had told us about him when she had visited us in the plastic apartment, and he was still, more than two months after he had gotten his heart, waiting for a clear biopsy so he could leave the hospital.

Transplants weren't allowed to visit in each other's rooms, and the only one I'd actually met had been Randy, walking in the hall with his parents and his nurse, but on the whole though, at the end of almost a week, I was feeling very well acquainted with ICU. I didn't stare with horror anymore as I passed rooms filled with intimidating machinery and unidentifiable bodies. I didn't flinch at the moans, groans, and gasping coughs, and I even knew that when you passed a room where a nurse appeared to be beating a patient to death, she wasn't; she was aiding in the emission of mucus. I had become a seasoned veteran.

One morning, I said hi at the nurses' station, deposited Sam's popsicle supply in the freezing compartment of the ICU refrigerator, and didn't even stare at the heavily garbed transplant I saw approaching as I left the diet kitchen. A transplant outside "its" room in ICU is an odd sight; it wears exactly what its visitors wear inside and, in addition, wheels along its IV pole with bottles and pacemaker attached. Its gait, known at Stanford as the ATG shuffle, is equally peculiar. Also, a transplant never ventures forth without its nurse.

Terry seldom left his room, I knew, and then only by wheelchair to go to X-ray, so I was just about to call, "Hi, Randy," when I saw that the nurse smiling and beckoning at me was Lynn. My composure vanished, and I tore down the hall to hug my own personal transplant, out in the world for the first time.

"Hello there, Mum," said Sam benevolently. "Come and walk with us. It's time I met everybody."

Like a dowager duchess calling on the poor, he made his progress, stopping and knocking at various doors on his way along the hall. Between doors he would fill me in on the exact condition of the patient within. Since this was his first outing, how he knew precisely who was who and where remains a mystery to me.

"Hi, Terry," he yelled cheerfully into the first door. "It's me, Sam. I'm out walking."

There was only a muted grunt in reply, and as we departed Sam remarked, "Terry's not very friendly, but I guess I wouldn't be either if I was as old as he is. He's over fifty, Mum, and Lynn says that's awfully old for a transplant. He smoked too," he added ominously, looking at me, "but, geez, he hasn't even rejected. You'd think he'd feel pretty good about the whole thing, but Lynn says he doesn't even want to start physical therapy. God, I wish they'd send his dumbbells down to my room."

"Don't complain," Lynn said. "You're out walking, aren't you? One thing at a time." We reached another port of call.

There was an "Oops, sorry" from Sam as he pushed open the door to reveal a patient quite obviously in extremis, and he didn't knock on any others until we'd crossed the hall into the self-care section and found Cobbie's room.

I heard a vigorous, thoroughly western voice answer Sam's greeting with a "Hey there, Sam. Great to see you out. Heard a lot about you. How're you doing?" Standing on my tiptoes in the doorway, peering around Sam, I saw a man sitting on the edge of the bed who might well have been a tackle for one of Sam's pro football teams — except for his legs, that is. They were scrawny below the knees, hideously swollen above, and a dark bluish purple over all.

"Look at me," he said. "Twenty-two straight nights of ATG. I hope they don't get that fierce with you, Sam."

Lynn giggled. "We won't, Cobbie. We're going to keep him off beer," and after we'd left the doorway, she said: "Did you see that little refrigerator on the wall across from his bed? He'd get a clear biopsy much quicker if he didn't have so much beer in it."

"I wish I had one just like it, just as full," Sam said wistfully.

A transplant was being done that morning, and at some point on our tour Lynn pointed out the closed door of the room where he was going to be. "He must be a very brave man," she said. "He's here all alone, and usually they won't accept transplants if they haven't got family backup. His wife couldn't leave her job because they have two kids she has to support."

"But where did he wait for his heart?" Sam asked, and when Lynn said it was at the VA hospital, all alone, he shook his head. "Geez" was all he said, but he didn't knock on any more doors until we got to Randy's.

"Hi, Randy, what's up?" he called in. "I thought you'd be out walking by this time. What'd ya have, a big night last night or something? C'mon, my walk'll be over by the time you get gowned up." Peering around Sam again, I got my first good look at the youngest transplant Stanford had ever done. He was sitting on the edge of his bed, talking to his mother and father. He looked awfully little and awfully young, and like Sam he was desperately thin. Under a shock of brown hair, his face was woebegone.

He smiled, though, and in a deep southern accent said, "Hey there, Sam, I can't; I'm rejectin'. My biopsy just came back and I can't leave the room anymore. I can't even do any physical therapy till I stop."

Sam shook his head. "Randy," he said, "it must be those pajamas you're wearing. That's gotta be what did it. You scared your heart!"

There wasn't any pause at all. "Well, at least I have some pajamas, Sam. Your nurses say you don't even own any. Down here at this end of the hall, we got a little class," and the two of them went at it back and forth until Lynn called a halt.

"You two! It's bad enough listening to you on the telephone. It's probably a good thing you can't leave your room, Randy. ICU will be a disaster area if the two of you ever get out in the hall together."

Randy's mother obviously agreed with her. "And to think

272

I told Randy to be quiet around you, Sam," she drawled. "I'd seen you at clinic before you got your heart, and you looked to me like the kind of boy who couldn't stand shoutin'. That was before I heard you on the phone. After that I said, 'Randy, you make all the noise you want around that boy. He's worse than you are!' "

We all acted as if there were nothing wrong at all, but Sam didn't say a word after we left Randy's room until he got back into bed, and it was plain that his joy in his outing was gone.

"I hope to hell he doesn't have a bad rejection," he said. "God, he's just a kid."

For Sam, though, it was too early to worry about rejection. His heart was just a week old when Rozzie called to say she couldn't stand one more minute of not knowing what a miracle looked like and was coming to California to view it. When I protested at the expense, she sepulchrally produced her irrefutable last word — "I talked to Mother, and she says . . ." — and ended the discussion.

Sam himself was ecstatic at the prospect of being viewed.

"What does Aunt Roz look like?" everyone asked.

"Like Mum," Sam said every time. "You seen one, you seen 'em both," and so, encountering Rozzie in the hallway as she arrived in ICU, Judy greeted her with "Oh, you must be Aunt Roz!"

"And you," Rozzie said, with a broad smile and without batting an eye, "must be Judy. Aunt Vic told me all about you over the phone."

I could never have replied that way, being vastly more reserved and lacking in savoir faire, but there were no more "Mrs. Pooles" after that, and in ICU the reunited Snoop Sisters became universally known as Aunt Roz and Aunt Vic.

273

Rozzie was just as confused and awkward gowning up for the first time as Parker and I had been. "Is it me, or is this very complicated?" she asked with some annoyance, fumbling down her back for the elusive ties that held the gown together. "Does it always take this long? I want to see Sam," and when the last glove was finally pulled on, she almost ran through the door of his room. She started to rush toward him and stopped dead in her tracks. There was an audible gasp.

"Say-am," she quavered, "you look just like Jesus Christ!"

That thought had crossed my mind too, but it had seemed sacrilegious, and I'd decided that I was probably getting carried away with all the miracle business. Looking at him again, though, I could not deny that he certainly bore a startling resemblance to Our Lord.

While he was sick nothing had grown, neither nails, nor beard, nor hair, but one short week of blood circulation had changed all that. His hair was already hanging luxuriantly about his shoulders, evidence of a golden beard was appearing, and, while it might well be argued that it wasn't spiritual fervor that lit up his eyes, it couldn't be denied that they glowed. The side effect of prednisone that Sam's vanity dreaded most was the chipmunk cheeks, but the medicine had yet to fill out his face, and he remained hollow of cheek and sunken of eye.

"Jesus Christ," she said again with solemn wonder, and the heart transplant murmured, "I know."

Before Rozzie came I had chiefly relied on Sam and the nurses to keep me up to date with the goings-on in ICU, but I should have remembered that information never gets to Rozzie secondhand. Gowning up to come into the room the very first day she was there, she learned from the horse's mouth, so to speak, that the mood swings of prednisone were not always — like Sam's — up. Terry's wife was dressing to go into her husband's room next door at the same time, and she looked so anguished that Rozzie asked her if everything was all right.

"Nothing's right," the woman said in a voice that verged on a sob. "Everything's awful, and it's all my fault. I guess Terry didn't really want the heart and he only came out here for my sake and the children's. If he has to die, I just hope it's soon because he's so disagreeable I can't stand it much longer."

Distressing as that information was, however, it paled by comparison with what Rozzie picked up the next day. I had just come out of Sam's room and was ungowning when I spotted her sitting with a young blond girl. The hallway outside Sam's room broadened into the inner waiting room of ICU, and Rozzie leapt to her feet when she spotted me and rushed toward me looking desperate.

"Oh, Aunt Vic," she whispered to me, indicating the girl with a jerk of her head, "she wants to meet the mother of the eighteen-year-old transplant. She thought I was you."

The girl was following Rozzie, and when she reached us she said to me, "I'm a friend of the donor, Mrs. Poole."

I stared at her. Lois had told Parker and me that Sam's heart had come from a seventeen-year-old boy who had been killed in a motorcycle accident not far from Stanford, but that was all. Knowing how Sam felt about his new heart, I hadn't even told him that. I couldn't seem to pull myself together enough to ask the girl how she knew about us. I just stood there.

"Oh, I'm not really here to see your son," she explained. "My father's a patient in ICU. But they told us in school assembly yesterday that Joey's heart had gone to an eighteen-year-old boy at Stanford, and I told the other kids I'd try to see what he looked like."

I finally managed to speak. "He's just about to come out of his room for a walk, but you mustn't say anything about knowing the donor. We're not supposed to know anything about it."

"Oh, I wouldn't," she exclaimed, "but, oh, Mrs. Poole, Joey loved sports so."

I nodded. "Sam does too," I said, and she started to go back to her seat. Suddenly she stopped and turned.

"Mrs. Poole," she said, "there's just one thing. Joey had an awful lot of girls." Finally I could breathe.

"His heart couldn't be in a better place, my dear," I said with a genuine smile just as Sam came out of his room with Lynn.

Even masked, gowned, and bonneted, he quite plainly hadn't lost his charms, and after he'd said hi and started off down the hall with Lynn, the girl tugged at my arm.

"He's handsome," she whispered. "I'll tell all the kids at school tomorrow."

"Rozzie," I hissed, as we joined the heart transplant parade, "you're not to make any more friends."

"I couldn't help it," she hissed back. "The girl told me they had an assembly one day and prayed for Joey, and the next day they had another and prayed for Sam."

In truth it wasn't Rozzie's fault that a half hour later we ran into Rick Taylor, the backup recipient for Sam's heart, but it seemed too much for one day. He and his wife were just coming out of the cafeteria as Rozzie and I went in, and he smiled at me and asked, "How's Sam doing?"

I remember thinking, How does he know who I am? and

then, suddenly, He must have been watching us that day in admissions just the way we were watching him, and the most dreadful wave of guilt swept over me.

With tears in my eyes, I said, "Oh, Rick, he's just fine, and the note you wrote him the night before he had the operation made all the difference in the world. Thank you," and to my surprise he leaned down from his great height and kissed my cheek.

"We're going back to Sam's room, and we're not leaving it again," I said to Rozzie, and we spent the rest of the day collecting our nerves and composing a poem we hoped would brighten Randy's term in solitary. We thought we did rather well.

"To Randy from Aunts Vic and Roz," we wrote:

> *Do not feel that you're alone*
> *For you have got your prednisone!*
> *On Coke there seems to be a ban,*
> *But, cheer up, you've got Imuran.*
> *And though you yearn for fat, not lean,*
> *You still have lovely Persantine.*
> *The Stanford dance of Dr. B*
> *Is called the shuffle ATG.*
> *So don't despair flat on your back —*
> *Spruce up your life with Titralac!*
> *The blues you'll gaily be combattin'*
> *While sucking on your Mycostatin;*
> *And, oh, those Stanford mouthwash kisses*
> *Are irresistible to misses.*
> *If you can't live a Life of Sin*
> *Console yourself with Coumadin!*
> *Remembering the Shumway Fix*

To cure your ills is called Lasix,
You will, at end of day, find solace
In swallowing your daily Colace.

Keeping Rozzie from socializing, however, is a losing battle. Looking neither to the right nor to the left myself, I went to get Sam a popsicle, and when I got back to the room Dr. Baumgartner was telling Rozzie that his wife was about to have a baby, and Rozzie was telling him that she would have to knit it a sweater. Life was very quiet after she went home.

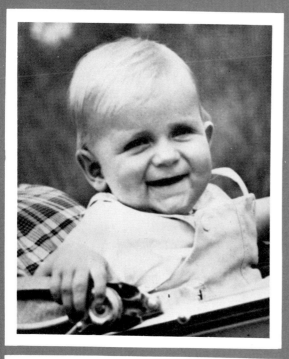

Sam at seven months, courtesy of Great-Aunt Esther Wright

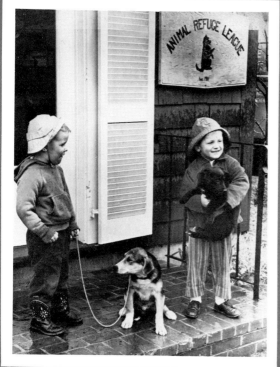

Freddie Gremmer, Sam (right) and friends

Sam and Alix,
1968

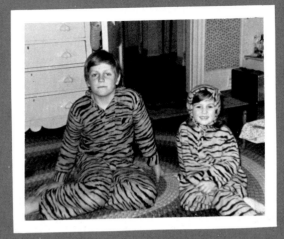

Old Number 71,
Kent Varsity
football, 1975

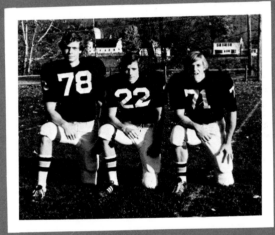

The mother and
Tina at the
Bicentennial
bash

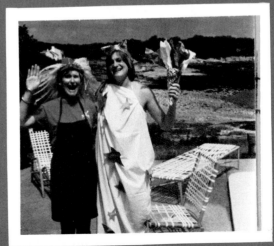

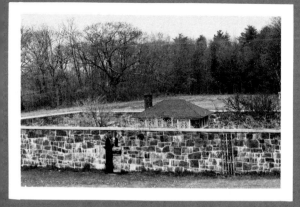

The Tea House

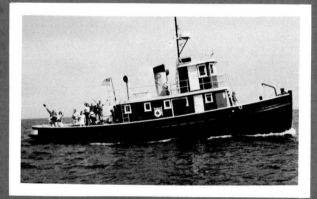

M.V. <u>Victoria</u>

Sam, on the
M.V. <u>Victoria</u>'s
maiden voyage,
September 1976

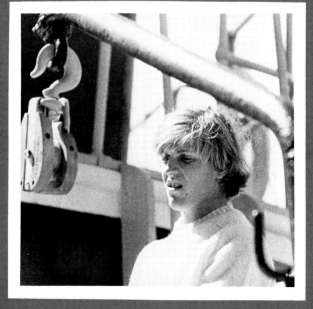

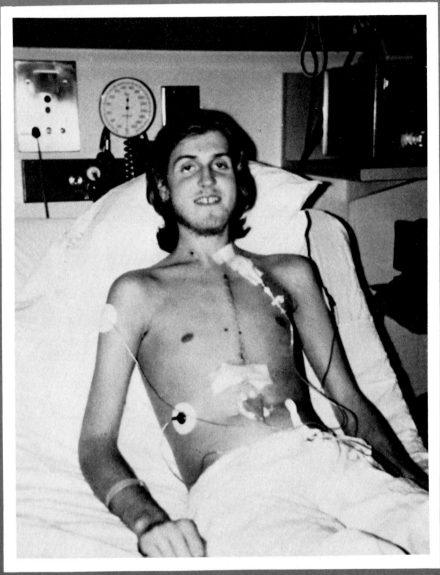

Sam, about three weeks after
the operation

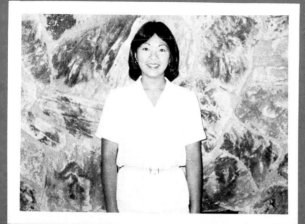

SAM'S NURSES

Lynn

Judy

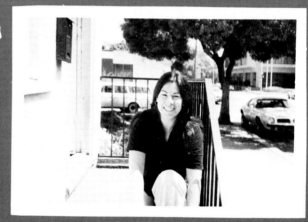

Kathy

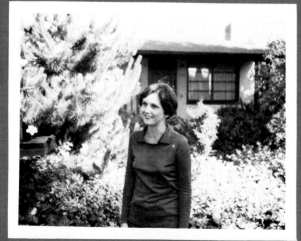

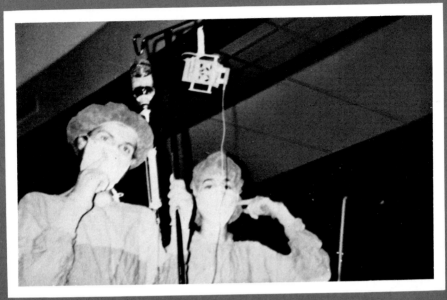

Sam (left) and Randy on their first walk
down the hall together

Sam with beer awarded by Dr. Baumgartner
after pacemaker installation

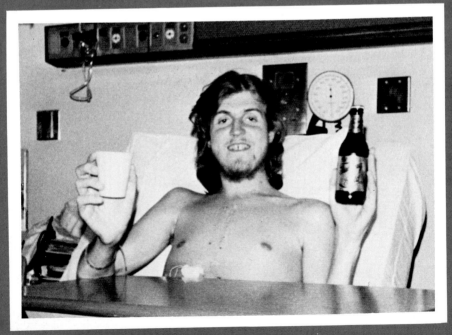

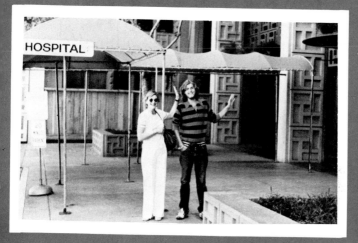

Leaving Stanford University Medical Center, April 3, 1977

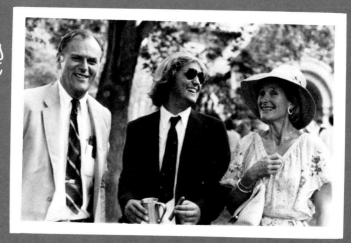

Sam graduating from Kent, May 1978

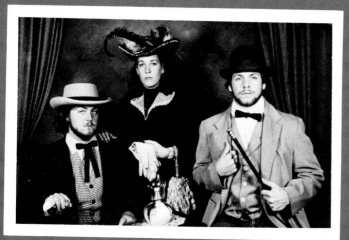

Heart Transplant 120 (left) with Stanford friend and the lady known as Claire

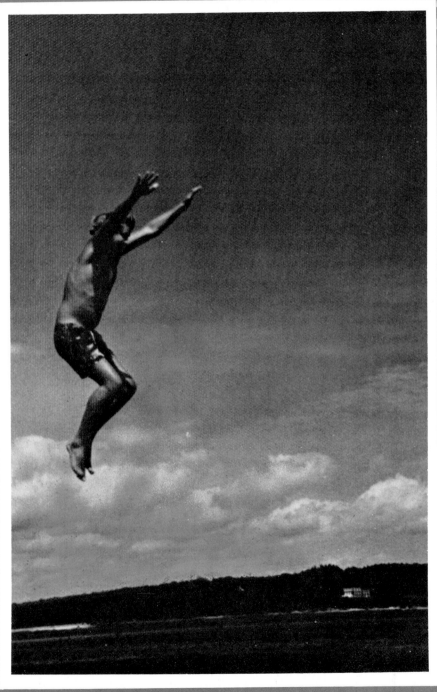

The first transplant to jump off the roof of a tugboat's pilothouse

Chapter Eleven
Sam had his first biopsy ten days after he got his heart, and it was clear, just as Randy's first one had been. There was no sign that he was rejecting at all.

The process of a biopsy sounded horrible to me. A thin tube was slipped through a tiny incision in the jugular vein and snaked down into the heart. The tube had tiny pincers at the end, and they snipped off a tiny piece of the transplanted heart. The tissue was then extracted, treated, and examined under an electron microscope for signs that a rejection was getting under way. A biopsy, I was told, could detect rejection well before the outward and visible effects appeared, and the invention of the process by a Stanford doctor had made a big difference in heart transplant statistics. Both Lynn and Judy had said that in the old days a rejection could be out of control before anyone even knew it was beginning.

Sam's first biopsy took a long time. The news came out of the operating room that Dr. Baumgartner was having a hard time getting the tube snaked down, but when Sam finally reappeared at his door on a stretcher he was the picture of nonchalance.

"Nothing to it; it's a breeze," he commented, as if he'd done the whole thing himself.

He was freed from the nightly torment of shots after that, and Dr. B told him there would be no more ATG until he rejected.

"And there's always the possibility you might not, Sam, you know," Judy said. "Two transplants never rejected at all," and I, who had made a lifetime policy of never looking on the bright side, threw caution to the winds and decided that Sam would become the third.

Only the return of his migraines marred his recovery, and they were cured in short order and forever by a violet-eyed nurse who substituted for Lynn one weekend. Her name was Kathy, and she had a crisp tongue and a succinct way of putting things.

He had a terrible seven-hour migraine the first day she was on with him, and the next morning, when I opened his door, I saw that the shades were still down and Sam only a mound under the bedcovers.

"Is it a bad one?" I whispered to her. The violet eyes opened wide, and the nurse drew herself up to her full five-foot height.

"Do you think you're dealing with an average, run-of-the-mill-type nurse from Elsewhere General?" she demanded. "I'll have you know I never allow my patients to suffer twice from the same complaint. 'Cure them,' I always say, 'or — ' " There was a significant pause while I quailed above her, and finally, with a regal wave of her arm toward the mound under the covers, she announced, "I have cured this particular one.

"Sam," she went on to explain, "is not a morning person. His headaches come from having to do things he doesn't like to do early in the day. I'm writing orders that he should never be touched before ten."

"Make it eleven," came a grunt from under the rumpled covers of the unmade bed; and Kathy, the substitute nurse, became a familiar fixture in Sam's room.

"I must have flipped," she said. "I loathe transplants," but she joined me in deciding that Sam was going to be the third transplant not to reject.

"A Fijian and a black haven't," she said, "why not a WASP? I hate WASPs on general principles, but Sam's such a nice one, and it would give the doctors something more to research."

The now-migraineless heart transplant didn't waste a minute worrying about whether he'd reject or not. He was too busy. "I gotta exercise; I gotta get some muscle back" became his motto as he strode down the halls, and Lynn, or Judy, or Kathy, and I followed him through every nook and cranny of Stanford, even past the POSITIVELY NO ADMITTANCE signs that marked every entrance to the vast new wing the hospital was building. By the end of a week, we had to trot to keep up with him, and he had begun to complain wistfully that what he really needed was fresh air.

"I just wish I could touch something green and growing again," he said, yet once allowed outside he didn't even glance at a tree or flower. His ATG shuffle turned into a hundred-yard dash, and, with Lynn and me in hot pursuit, he sped like a homing pigeon for the doctors' parking lot — a peculiar sight with his gloved hand clutching his IV pole, his bonnet and mask askew, and his gown flapping in the breeze. What he wanted to savor was Porsches, and not until he had counted three 928s, five 911s, and four 914s did he consent to withdraw to a sunny bench near the fountains.

I enjoyed every minute of Sam's newborn life. Even though Lynn complained that his was the smallest room in ICU and that, with the impedimenta that seemed to attach itself to him, he needed a suite, I wouldn't have swapped it for the Waldorf Towers. The whole wall opposite the door was a window, and above the deep window ledge where Sam's belongings were piled high, and where I loved to sit, the daisy-splattered shades were bright and cheerful. The walls had become a collage of get-well cards, and below the chart of medications, Lynn had tacked up the "I Left My Heart in San Francisco" T-shirt she'd bought for Sam on a day off. The biopsies that began to be scheduled one right after the other as the time grew ripe for rejection were the only reminder that things could still go wrong.

Sam's second biopsy didn't show any rejection cells at all either, and, as if that weren't enough cause for me to be euphoric, Lois Christopherson's prediction came true: all his brain needed was a little blood circulation to get it working again.

Out of the blue one night he said, "I wish I'd brought Grampa's Robert Service poems out here. It'd be kinda nice to have you read to me at night." I dashed to the nearest bookstore and bought not only Service but every book of familiar poetry I could find. Cremating Sam McGee and wrecking the Hesperus became integral parts of our evenings, but writing remained another matter.

"Tomorrow," he'd groan when I'd tell him he ought to write a thank-you note, and when pressed: "You do it, Mum. You oughta keep busy." But on Valentine's Day there had been an envelope in the mailbox at the plastic, addressed to me in handwriting I hadn't seen since November. The card inside said, "I love you — *Sam*," and I'd sniffed with happiness all the way upstairs to the apartment.

I would have done better to pursue my lifetime philosophy of looking on the dark side. The day after his third biopsy, Dr. Baumgartner appeared in his room just as we were getting ready to go out for a walk.

"I'm sorry, partner," he said to Sam. "You're rejecting. The results just came down from the lab, and I'm afraid we've got to ground you."

Kathy was on duty, and she said, "See, Sam, I told you WASPs never have any luck," but other than being incarcerated in his room and having to endure ATG again, rejection didn't seem to bother him at all at the beginning.

It bothered his nurses much more. He was put on such huge doses of immunosuppressants to counteract the rejection that they were in terror of his picking up an infection.

"If anyone walked into this room with a cold sore now, it could turn into bubonic plague for the kid," Kathy said.

Lynn became phobic about germs. She scrubbed his room and scoured it, and she delighted Sam by chasing Dr. Shumway, who never gowned up to survey his patients, out the door with a mop.

Sanitized and smiling, Sam held court in his chamber. A somewhat dramatic friend of mine had written him a letter describing the agonies of her own chest surgery, and, quoting from it, he took to answering knocks on the door with a cheery "Welcome to the world of pain, and fear, and aloneness." It was a nice world.

Lynn talked him into hooking a rug, and, although he protested that he felt like "one of Santa's goddamned elves" and it was going "to ruin his image," he hooked and looped away with a will those first days of his rejection. A beautiful blond began knocking at his door at least three times a day. When the nurses and I began to speculate as to her intentions, he calmly said "Rape," with his customary leer.

He talked Judy into borrowing her father's Polaroid camera, and I got used to entering his room to find him, IV pole, tubes, wires, and all, trying to look statuesque and muscular with Judy laughing too hard to snap the shutter.

"Hurry up," he'd plead, "I can't keep my bicep out much longer."

I got even more used to two words I'd heard ever since he got his heart but hadn't paid much attention to before: "voltage" and "rosettes." They suddenly became the chief concern of every day. The EKG given twice daily determined Sam's voltage, and up was where it ought to be and wasn't; a daily blood test and clinical processing gave the count of rosettes, and down was where they should be and weren't.

Every two or three days there was another biopsy, and with every one a stronger rejection pattern was recorded, but the nurses were still very reassuring. A fluoroscopic view of Sam's heart was taken each time he had a biopsy to measure the distance between two metal clips that had been implanted in the heart during surgery. As long as those clips didn't begin to spread apart, they said, there was nothing to worry about.

"And if they do?" I asked nervously.

Well, that would mean that the heart was enlarging and not able to pump properly. But Sam's clips were still just where they ought to be. "And that's where they're gonna stay," the transplant said firmly.

Randy had been transplanted ten days before Sam and had been rejecting strongly for eleven. The news that began to drift down the hall from his room wasn't reassuring at all and made me very edgy about what was in store for Sam.

"Rejecting like a bandit" was one nurse's description of how Randy was coming along. "God, how that skinny kid's legs can take one more night of shots I don't know," despaired another. Finally Judy came into Sam's room one night looking anguished.

"Dr. Baumgartner just told Randy's parents that it looks as though this heart isn't going to work for Randy. He thinks he's going to have to have a second transplant," she said.

I remember thinking, God couldn't be that cruel; and reading the poem about a boy's will being the wind's will to Sam after his shots that night, it was all I could do to keep myself from saying, "Screw you, Longfellow," out loud.

Sam and Randy had been talking back and forth on the phone at least three times a day, comparing notes on "solitary," starvation, and shots, but the day after Judy told us about the second heart, there were no calls at all, and it was no comfort to hear from the nurses the list of transplants who had had to have a replacement.

"It's the youngest ones who reject the worst," Lynn said, but suddenly — just as suddenly as it had begun — Randy's rejection ended. By nightfall the next day, his voltage had gone up, his rosettes had gone down, and when I got to the hospital after supper, Sam was conducting a raucous telephone call.

"Boy, those pajamas really got you into big trouble, Randy. I told you, ya gotta play it cool with a new heart — nothing startling — subdued colors for us transplants."

So Randy was safe for the moment; and the new transplant, Fred, who had been done the day Sam took his first walk in the hall, was reportedly doing wonderfully well. He was a police detective from Florida, and Lynn had been right in her surmise that he must be a very brave man. Whenever Sam knocked on his door to say hello, Fred seemed as nonchalant and cheerful as if he were in for minor surgery and not thirty-five hundred miles from home without a soul to visit him. He gave everybody a lift, but you could never breathe entirely easily in ICU.

Next door to Sam, things were going from bad to worse with Terry, the older transplant. He was desperately sick with a lung infection. And as often as I tried to tell myself that I was imagining it, Sam himself was not where he had been a week before. He abandoned his rug hooking and lay most of the day quietly listening to his FM radio; Judy's Polaroid sat filled with unused film on the window ledge; and our days became reminiscent enough of the long quiet ones before he got his heart to make me yearn for it to be time for Parker to come back.

Everything started to go wrong. Not because of his rejection and for no apparent reason, Sam's heartbeat without the pacemaker became frighteningly slow. The technician who usually did the EKGs was off one day, and the girl who took his place turned off his pacemaker.

Kathy was on duty, and after a minute or so Sam said to her, "I feel kinda dizzy." A minute later he said, "I feel like I'm going to pass out," and Kathy took his pulse and gasped.

"I'll just bet you do," she said. "Turn on the pacemaker," she directed the technician.

"But Dr. Baumgartner wants the EKG done with the pacemaker off," the girl protested.

Kathy switched it on herself. "Then Dr. Baumgartner

will be missing one transplant," she snapped. "The kid's heart almost stopped beating."

His heartbeat began to affect my own one morning as I sat quietly in the chair next to his bed, writing a letter to Tina in England. Sam had barely said a word since I got there, and I wrote, "There is very little news today, but we are —" and then I just happened to look over at Sam and noticed that one of the wires that led from the pacemaker and usually hooked into his stomach was instead attached to nothing.

"Shouldn't that wire go somewhere?" I asked him, and he started to peer down at it over his chest, but before he could even answer, the nurse filling in during Lynn's lunch break leapt to her feet. She took one horrified look at the wire, grabbed a long needle from the supply tray, and jabbed it so quickly into Sam's stomach that he couldn't even flinch.

He and I were both staring as she attached what looked exactly like miniature jumper cables for a car battery first to the needle and then to the pacemaker wire. Simultaneously Sam started jolting up and down.

"Turn it off," he gasped. "I'm getting shocks!"

But the nurse just cried, "I can't. You have to have the pacemaker going," and with that she fled to the door and yelled down the hall for the charge nurse.

"And page Dr. Baumgartner too," she cried, before running back to Sam.

The charge nurse deftly replaced the needle and the cable farther away from the disconnected wire in his stomach and explained with awesome competence that Sam had been short-circuiting. "You had the needle too close to the other outlet," she said.

After Dr. Baumgartner came and checked Sam over, all

he did was burst out laughing. "I guess what you need is a little agony every morning to get that heartbeat going, partner," he said. "You're going faster than the pacemaker" — which was consoling, but I had to finish my letter to Tina outside.

"I have retreated to the coffee cup and the sunshine to regroup my nerves," I wrote. "If there are many more days like this, I fear, as we say at Stanford, I shall become a donor."

Toward the end of that week of catastrophe, Terry died. No amount of antibiotics had been able to cope with his lung infection, and for days it had been no secret that there was little hope for him. I was still startled, though, when Kathy came into Sam's room and said bluntly: "Sam, Terry's just died. I'm telling you right now so you won't hear rumors about it, but you mustn't think the same thing will happen to you. Terry's situation was completely different from yours. He was a lot older, and it was harder for him, and he didn't want the heart the way you did. Now you, Sam — nobody's going to get that heart away from you."

I wished her eyes looked as confident as the words sounded, but when I looked over at Sam it was plain that he wasn't even thinking about himself.

"Poor Terry," he said. "Poor guy, he had an awful rough time."

On the way home that night I saw Rick Taylor's wife sitting alone in one of the waiting rooms on the floor below ICU, and one look at her face told me that it wasn't because a heart had finally come along for Rick. She looked up from her knitting when she saw me, though, and smiled.

"Everything okay?" I asked.

The smile faded. "He's got pneumonia," she said. "They

took him off the transplant waiting list this afternoon."

"What a rotten goddamned business," I kept muttering to myself all the way home, and back in the plastic apartment I took Lynn's Hawaiian calendar off the wall and looked at the list I'd made of the people who'd gotten hearts since Thanksgiving.

Burpee:	Thanksgiving Day — Died Jan. 25
Cobbie:	Dec. 7 — Out of ICU Feb. 2
Terry:	Jan. 7 —
Randy:	Jan. 25 —
Sam:	Feb. 3 —
Fred:	Feb. 8 —

Died Feb. 25, I wrote after Terry's name, and then, looking at the list, I slapped my hand over my mouth.

"Oh, God," I moaned. "If it's every other one, Sam isn't going to make it."

There was no comfort in looking at Sam anymore. As hard as I tried not to "trouble trouble," I couldn't avoid noticing that his cheeks weren't pink anymore, or his toes warm, and, rejection symptoms aside, there was no denying that his legs were a shambles. Almost as discolored as Cobbie's had been after his twenty-two-day ordeal, swollen above the knees, and covered with angry red needle marks, they hurt me just to look at them, and Lynn started taking the afternoon and evening shifts when Judy was off duty so that no novice would ever have to give Sam the ATG. Listening to me read had seemed to help him get his mind off the pain at the beginning of his rejection, but no longer. He never complained during the shots or after them, but lay twisting and turning in bed, biting his lip and gingerly rubbing his thighs in an effort to get the ATG moving, while

Judy or Lynn watched him with eyes that were almost as tormented as his.

At that point Lynn found out that Randy's nurses were trying what they called meditation therapy with him. It seemed to help. Having learned the magic words one said to induce meditation, and having practiced one entire evening at home with her fiancé, she was ready for Sam when it was time for shots the next night.

She turned out all the lights in the room except the dim one near the entrance and directed Sam to lie back on the pillows.

"You are in an elevator, Sam," she said, in a hushed dull voice entirely empty of its usual happy lilt. "You are going down, down, down to a faraway place where you are very happy. You are so comfortable; you are so happy; you are so at peace that you can hardly move. You hear nothing, you see nothing, you feel nothing, you are so peaceful, so happy . . ."

On and on she went, her voice guiding him, but it wasn't meditation therapy she was practicing; it was hypnosis, and when I woke up the shots were all over, and Sam was not amused in the least.

"Mu-um," he protested, "it's supposed to be for me. I'm the one who gets the shots," but despite my behavior, it did seem to help the pain.

Nothing, however, seemed able to check his rejection, and his fifth biopsy cost me my last consoling thought. The fluoroscopic view of his heart showed that the clips were moving apart; there was no doubt that his heart was enlarging.

When I picked Parker up at the airport the next day, March 26, I didn't even ask him what he thought about my staying in California until Sam was out of danger. I simply told him I was.

As I knew he would, he went through the car roof. "You're not playing this thing by the numbers, Victoria," he roared. "We agreed that we'd each take three weeks here and three weeks at home. It's your turn to go home, and it's mine to be in the apartment."

"Fine," I said. "Stay in the apartment. I'll go to the Holiday Inn," and that startled him so he never said another word all the way to the hospital.

After he saw Sam and talked to Dr. Baumgartner, I think he must have understood why I'd been so determined to stay. Although he didn't say then that he agreed with my decision, he did at least stop calling me Victoria. The report wasn't good. Sam's voltage was still dropping, his rosettes were still climbing, and an echogram showed that fluid was building up around his heart.

Sam had been rejecting almost two weeks by then, and a day or so after Parker came, the two of us took a dismal walk, trying to cheer each other up. It was a forebodingly gray overcast afternoon, but it hadn't rained a drop for weeks, and the grass was brown, lying in dusty clumps on the hard-packed earth. The footpaths were even dustier and harder packed, and the huge eucalyptus trees that surround the university looked dead. Scurrying into their dusty holes, even the little gray ground squirrels, the companions I'd delighted in on many a solitary walk, looked mangy and diseased.

"His voltage was up a little last night," Parker said.

"And his rosettes went down a little too, so that's good," I said, about five ground squirrels later.

"I wish he felt better, though," he said when we were back on the hospital grounds.

"Me too," I said.

At the door of the hospital he said, "I'm glad you stayed," and I knew that he was just as frightened as I was.

We met Dr. Baumgartner outside Sam's door, dressing to go in the room, and he looked worried and exhausted.

"We just got the results of the latest biopsy," he said, "and the rejection is finally resolving. That explains why the voltage went up and the rosettes were down."

I stopped tying my gown and I remember thinking for a split second, Oh, how wonderful! But the look on Dr. Baumgartner's face kept me from saying it.

"I'm afraid I have some awfully bad news for you," he said. "I think we've got to start looking for a new heart for Sam. This one's got a bad gallop sound now. It's inflamed, too, and so enlarged it's not handling the fluid. His weight's gone way up, and that's a sure sign of fluid buildup."

My heart sank, but, clutching at straws, I said: "But you said the rejection was resolving. Won't that clear it up?"

He shook his head sadly. "I'm afraid not. You see, it looks as if the heart will be permanently damaged by the time it does fully resolve. Sam would be right back where he was with his old heart. We couldn't leave him that way," and he pulled his mask up over his mouth and nose and went into Sam's room with Parker and me trailing behind.

He walked over to Sam's bed, felt the pulse in his ankles, and then — and I couldn't believe he was doing it — looked him straight in the eye and told him just what he'd told us.

"We can keep you going a long time with this heart while we look for another one, Sam," he finally finished, "but if things haven't changed by tomorrow night, I guess we'd better start looking."

Sam hadn't moved from the time Dr. Baumgartner started to speak, and his face hadn't changed expression.

He just lay there listening, and when Dr. Baumgartner had finished, he looked up at him and said quietly, "Okay, Dr. B."

That was all, but, after the meditation and the shots that night, he asked me to read him the Service poem we'd both loved because it made us think of Camp Bruin. My voice broke when I read

> . . . *and often I'll think of you, empty and black,*
> *Moose antlers nailed over your door:*
> *Oh, if I should perish my ghost will come back*
> *To dwell in you, cabin, once more.*

I was ashamed of myself, but I couldn't help it, and I tried to pretend I was keeping my head down to look for another poem.

"Hey, Mum," I heard Sam say, and when I looked up at him, tears and all, he was smiling at me — the most tender, gentle smile I've ever seen.

"Hey, you guys, don't *you* get upset," he said, turning his head to smile at Parker on the other side of the bed. "All along the great thing you did was never making it seem like you were worried. I knew you were, but if you'd gotten all upset or acted that way, it would have made me feel awful. It was nice that way — we all knew, but nobody showed it. Don't worry about this thing. I can handle it."

I couldn't speak, but Parker said, "Sammy, you're something else."

"Look, Dad," Sam said, "right at the beginning I said I'd rather die doing something to try to get better than die just doing nothing. Way back last fall when I was at Kent and the migraines were so bad, I learned that the worse the pain got, the more I could take it. I mean, I'd go to class having a small migraine and I could get through it — like do my reading and stuff. I guess I learned then that when you feel terrible, no matter how bad it is, you adjust. No matter how bad things look, you adjust yourself to them and you get by, no matter what anybody thinks. It's like that with the shots, or taking the medicines, or even this thing with the heart. If I gotta, I gotta. I can handle it."

"How can he be like that?" I asked Parker when we were in bed that night. We were both so awed by Sam's courage that we'd hardly spoken since we left the hospital.

"He's goddamned brave, that's how," Parker said. "He's the bravest kid I've ever seen."

Having said that, neither of us was prepared to find Sam sobbing when we got to his room the next morning. "What is it?" I cried, running to the bed, but his face was buried in the pillows and he didn't answer.

The nurse who was with him picked up a letter that was lying next to him on the bed and handed it to me. Her name was Jessica, and she was a friend of Lynn's who'd taken care of Sam a lot, but I'd never seen her outside the room. All I knew of her face were her eyes. Usually they were as gentle as a doe's, but they were hard with anger now. I grabbed the letter.

It was another from my "world of pain, and fear, and aloneness" friend, and this time she said she understood Sam had turned into "a spoiled, crotchety, impatient patient." "My tentative sympathy to your mother," she had finished. It was ill-timed humor, but nothing worse than that, and I tried to make light of it.

"Oh, Sam," I said, "don't get upset over that. She's just trying to be funny. You know her," but he sat up and glared at me with a face contorted with anger.

"I haven't been that way," he sobbed. "I've never complained. Why would she say that?"

"Because she's crazy!" Parker bellowed so loudly that he startled me. I spun around to look at him. He was furious. "You write that goddamned woman today and tell her she's never to write Sam again," he snarled, so ferociously that Sam stopped sobbing and started to laugh.

"Go, Dad," he cheered, and the crisis was over.

That was the only laugh in Sam's room that morning. His voltage had plunged again, his weight was up even more from fluid, and his legs were so sore that Jessica had gotten an air mattress for his bed.

"I thought it might take some of the pressure off his legs," she said sadly, "but it doesn't seem to do much good."

Parker and I sat silently in our chairs with all the resignation of pretransplant days. If he has to have another heart, he has to have one, I kept saying to myself. It often happens. They told us so. They'll find him one, and we'll start all over again.

And that was my frame of mind when Jessica asked Dr. Baumgartner if he thought Lasix given intravenously rather than orally might help Sam. "At least if he got rid of some of the fluid, his heart wouldn't have to work so hard," she said, and when Dr. Baumgartner said it couldn't hurt, she emptied a syringe of Lasix into the shunt in Sam's neck.

About fifteen minutes later, Sam said, "I gotta pee," and in just such an inelegant manner did his second miracle begin. He peed through the afternoon, and he peed through the night, and he was still peeing triumphantly when Parker and I got to the hospital the next morning.

It was as simple as that, and when Dr. Baumgartner

came into the room that night he was wreathed in smiles.

"Well, partner," he said, "if you really like the heart all that much, I guess we'll have to let you keep it. It's looking good. Your voltage has gone sky-high, and the X-ray shows your heart's gone right back to normal."

I was so excited that I ran headlong out of the room, crashed into Lois Christopherson, the social-service worker, immaculately clad in a black wool coat, and threw both my arms around her. I wasn't even ashamed of myself until I stepped back and saw that I had smeared her with Erno's best makeup from collar to mid-sleeve.

When the results of the next biopsy came back two days later, Sam's first rejection was officially declared resolved, and although Dr. Baumgartner could still hear the gallop sound in the heart, he said he was sure it would disappear in time. Sam could leave his room, he could have a night off from shots, and, yes, he had earned a gin and tonic.

"Now will you go home?" Parker said to me, and I said yes and I did, but not before I saw Sam and Randy finally meet in the hall of ICU.

Mask to mask and bonnet to bonnet, they solemnly shook blue-gloved hands, and side by side, propelling their IV poles, with their nurses beside them and their parents trailing in their wake, they made a jubilant progress through ICU. The two long, bare legs beneath the gown of the transplant on the right ended in feet encased in untied Adidas, but the feet of the other transplant went unnoticed for the brilliance of the maroon, orange, and bright green paisley of his pajama bottoms. They were the four most beautiful legs in all the world.

Chapter Twelve

Not once in all the many years that Parker and I have been married had I been away from home for so long. A two- or three-week vacation produces quite enough havoc, and normally I am geared forty-eight hours ahead of my return for broken washing machines, jammed disposals, and recalcitrant repair men. As my plane approached Portland on the morning of March 6, I should properly have been thinking of future crises, but instead I was still wallowing in the glories of the past five weeks.

His wait, his operation, and a full-fledged rejection behind him, my heart transplant was happily sipping the first gin and tonic of his new life as I bade him farewell. For my part, regardless of the fact that I hadn't slept a wink on the red-eye special, I felt marvelous.

I had planned to sleep, but no sooner had I sat down in my seat than the man sitting next to me lost a lens out of his glasses. Flushed with the successes of the past few days, I replaced it for him with the skill of an optometrist.

He beamed at me. "I never talk to people on planes," he said.

I beamed back at him and said, "Neither do I," and we picked up our books, but it was almost impossible to concentrate.

Our seat was besieged by one flight attendant after another, all hoping that my companion had everything he wanted, and finally, after the captain himself had appeared, the man turned to me and said, "You must be wondering who I am."

I stared at him blankly, realizing that if I should have, I hadn't. He was a nice-looking man about my age, and there certainly had been something familiar about him, but I had put it down to his sports coat's being very Parkerish.

"Oh, dear," I said nervously, and because he was still looking at me, waiting for an answer, I was just about to add, "I'm terrible at faces," when I realized I'd seen the man on television. Remembering that everyone who had passed our seat had asked him how things were in San Francisco, I cried with genuine delight, "Oh, I know. You're the sheriff of San Francisco, the one who went to jail."

His face fell. "No, I'm not," he said, sounding dashed. "I'm George Moscone, the mayor," and after that, disregarding our earlier statements, we talked all night long.

He was a dear. He told me about his daughter, who was having to spend six weeks in bed because of an injury, and I told him about Sam, and when we parted in Atlanta at five o'clock in the morning we were friends.

"You must bring your son to visit me in San Francisco when he's out of the hospital," he said, and, although I knew I never would — and now sadly never can — meeting

"My Mayor," I decided, was just the way a triumphal trip ought to end.

I was supremely self-satisfied as I swept off the plane in Portland. There wasn't a speck or a spot on my traveling off-white, for a wonder my beige wide-brimmed hat sat on my head at just the proper angle, and my tan leather boots were undeniably natty. If Rozzie had been meeting my plane, she would have said, "Did you eat it with the feathers on, or did you pluck it first?"

But Rozzie didn't meet me; Dottie did, and one look at her face told me I had been away too long. My boots began to hurt. I pulled off my hat and dropped a cigarette ash on the coat.

"What's gone wrong?" I asked with dread.

"You'll see," she said ominously, and as I got out of the car at the Cape, I did. No lawn in Maine is attractive in March, but by the back door ours had become an abattoir. Wads of yellowish-brown coarse hair were strewn across the graying patches of remaining snow; here could be seen a hoof; there identified a shank bone.

"Dear God," I gasped. "What happened?"

"Don't waste your time getting upset out here," Dottie retorted. "Save it for what's inside."

Along with the deer, three of my best rugs had been victimized. Dottie had been scrubbing them all morning and the worst was gone, but it was obvious that venison was too rich a menu for a dog brought up on Alpo.

Being a wily deerslayer, it seemed, was a time-consuming effort, and Moriah was nowhere to be seen. "She took off again this morning before I'd found the rugs," Dottie said. "She evidently hasn't heard there's a limit on deer, but look at it this way" — with a sour smile she pointed to

299

the huge dark stain that spread evilly over the pink and blue wildflowers of the prized hooked rug in our bedroom — "your new house sure as hell looks lived in."

After the drama of the past five weeks, it was almost relaxing to be back on all fours with the ammonia bottle and the Spic and Span. As the days slipped by, I progressed cheerfully from rugs to woodwork and woolens, and with Sam in Parker's hands and the dog securely tied on a run, I began to worry as I should — and for the first time in ages — about the other children.

I began with Tina. Before she went back to England after Christmas, she had told Parker and me that she was going to give up her spring term there to help us with Sam.

"I'll go to summer school, I promise," she'd said, "but I know I can help you and Dad if I'm home, and I just can't stand being so far away when everything's so awful. Maybe by spring Sam will have his heart, and I can stay with him so you and Dad can have some time together."

Right then I had missed her too much to be objective. "Okay," I'd agreed, and she was to come home on April 7 to cheer up Parker on his birthday.

Just after Sam got his heart, though, she'd dropped another bombshell. A letter came saying that, before she did come home, she was going to tour Greece with Him.

"But, my darling child," I'd written back, "you hardly know him. How do you know he's not an ax murderer?"

The letter waiting for me at home wasn't the least bit consoling. "Don't worry, Mum," it said. "I've written and asked him if he was. I told him my mother wants to know."

Fortunately none of the other children seemed to require my motherly concern. After one look at Alix's round rosy face, the pediatrician burst out laughing at my request on

Sam's behalf that she have a chest X-ray. "Well, if you insist," he'd said, "but she certainly doesn't look like she's suffering from cardiomyopathy to me."

The news from California, too, despite the fact that I was on pins and needles before each phone call, was uniformly good. There wasn't a hint of infection, which is — next to rejection — the greatest dread of a heart transplant, and the gallop sound in Sam's new heart had vanished altogether. His heartbeat was a little slow at night, but the pacemaker was off in the daytime now, and the heart seemed to go great guns as long as he was up and around.

It turned out to be absolutely true that heart transplants don't panic easily. Someone had pulled out a chair from behind Sam by mistake just as he was about to sit down, and he had crashed — IV pole, pacemaker, and all — to the floor of the ICU waiting room.

"My heart never missed a beat," Sam exulted to me over the phone, "but poor old Dad almost went into cardiac arrest. We were ready to wheel him off to a donor room."

I'd barely been home a week before the report came that the shunt had been taken out of his neck and that, freed of the IV pole, he'd pedaled a whole mile on the stationary bike in the physical-therapy room. He wore the pacemaker now, on a belt around his waist.

Just hearing Sam's voice was magic, and after I hung up I'd always call Rozzie first and then, in order of age, Dottie, Malcolm and Ruthie, Pokie, and sometimes, throwing economy to the winds, Charlie in Hartford and tell it all over again. Being at home, poor Alix was a continual captive audience.

Everyone knew that Parker had fallen asleep in the relaxing class that had been started for the transplants to help them get through the ATG shots. And everybody knew that although Sam was running a fever, it was only from ATG and nothing to worry about, according to Dr. Baumgartner. What was to be worried about was his heartbeat. It was now slowing down drastically at night, but I told everyone what Kathy, succinct as always, had said.

"Nothing's really wrong. It's just that the kid dies when he goes to sleep. So maybe he will have to have a permanent pacemaker put in. It sure as heck beats being dead."

Everyone had heard that Parker, being Parker, had found the most glamorous-sounding apartment, right near the hospital, for Sam to recuperate in, with a swimming pool, a gymnasium, and tennis courts; and they all heard my unequivocal opinion that "there is just no one in the world like Parker Poole." Everyone politely hung on every word I said — even poor Ruthie, who was days overdue with the baby and had just cause to want to talk about her condition instead of Sam's.

Outside the family, awe was the general reaction. I didn't see many people, but when I did the first question everybody asked was, "Do you know whose heart it was?" and I said routinely, "It was a boy's who was killed in a motorcycle accident."

Only to Freddie Gemmer's parents did I tell the story about Rozzie's girl in ICU, and only once did I get upset by a question about the donor.

It came at a bad time, the day after I heard that Rick Taylor, the backup recipient for Sam's heart, had died of pneumonia. Sam had been close to tears when he told me. "He was only twenty-seven years old, Mum. He never had another chance," he said, and when I went to market the next morning I was still hearing him say it and remembering how Rick had bent down and kissed me.

I was certainly in no mood to face the friend I saw determinedly wheeling her cart down an aisle toward me. She always manages to say just the wrong thing at precisely the wrong moment, and, having trapped me in the noodles section, she said: "I've just been reading about Christiaan Barnard doing all this work with baboon hearts. Are you really sure Sam got a human one?"

I couldn't help myself. "Who gives a damn?" I snapped. "He's alive," and I grabbed my noodles and fled.

Answering other questions was fun. "Is he able to get out of bed yet? Is he going to have to be awfully careful?" people would ask.

I loved saying casually, "Well, right now he's only riding a bicycle and doing weight lifting at the hospital, but when I go back I have orders to bring out his bathing suits and two tennis rackets."

Only within the family did I mention the one rule for transplants that still seemed hard to imagine: that for the rest of his life, Sam would have to wear a mask in public places. It was a measure of how well he was getting along that I even thought about it at all. I would never have quibbled with anything Stanford said, but it did seem odd to think of Sam sitting in a bar with his friends with a hard blue plastic shield covering his nose and mouth. I wondered how he'd handle it.

At least to her own satisfaction, Rozzie had already solved that problem. "I'll have some designed for him at Gucci," she said. "They'll be marvelous. Everybody will want to wear them!"

All in all, though, the worst did seem to be behind us, and for the first time in my life I began to feel like an authority on something other than housecleaning. I must have been a dreadful bore. There wasn't a thing about cardiomyopathy or having a heart transplant I didn't think I knew. There wasn't a detail of what had happened or was happening to Sam that I couldn't recall at the drop of a hat, and I was glib with descriptions of when and where it had happened. It was only at night, lying in bed alone in the new bedroom with the corner windows open to the sea and the wind, that I admitted that I didn't know the whys for anything. Like the events of an endless crazy dream, everything had assumed vast importance, but it was all undifferentiated in my mind. Like a dream too it was impossible to sort out cause from effect, and even when I asked myself a question, my mind, like an improperly programmed computer, produced a fact that didn't answer anything:

Why did he push so hard last summer? (The first time I saw his chest pound was the night of the Tea House Party.)

If his heart fell apart when they took it out, what kept him alive? (Dr. Shumway said it was as thin as paper and spotted like a leopard's hide.)

If Freddie Gemmer hadn't come to the Cape to see me just before Parker came back from California, I might have gone on that way forever.

Lanky, slouching a little, with the shy sweet smile that says "I hope I'm not interrupting," he appeared one afternoon in the kitchen, surprising Moriah, who flew at him barking and then, seeing it was Fred, waggled around him apologetically.

It was Dottie's day off and I was ironing in the kitchen. Ruthie had finally had the baby, and, being Freddie, he sat down in a rocking chair with the dog at his feet and cheerfully and patiently endured all the news every new grandmother has to impart. He'd given up the eyeglasses he'd worn since childhood, and behind the contact lenses I still wasn't quite used to, his blue eyes looked genuinely interested in the fact that little Malcolm Augustus had weighed seven pounds and nine ounces and looked just like his father. His head nodded its mass of reddish gold curls with just the proper admiration at Ruthie's being clever enough to produce a baby on St. Patrick's Day, and it was only after it was plain that there was absolutely nothing more anyone could say about a three-day-old baby that he finally said, "How is Sam, Mrs. Poole?"

I looked up from my ironing, ready to let flow the usual flood of details, but, looking at him, I knew that wasn't what he really wanted to hear. He knew Sam too well to want that, and anyway he'd probably already heard it all directly.

"Freddie," I said — and it was the greatest relief to say it finally — "I know he's fine, and I know he's going to be able to cope with this, but what I don't know is why. I still don't know how he got through the awful mess. Sometimes I look back at the way he pushed himself last summer, and it seems as if he was trying to make himself sicker, and yet, when the only thing left was having the heart transplant, there was no way he wasn't going to live to get one."

"But that's Sam, Mrs. Poole," Freddie said without the slightest hesitation. "You gotta know that. He gets psyched up for things — games, or parties, or even bad things like this. He's always done it. The reason he pushed so hard last summer was to prove he was stronger than he was sick. The worse he felt, the harder he pushed. He told me a year ago that he had this thing about being sick. 'If you don't keep active, if you don't do anything, even if you're sick,' he told me, 'things are gonna get worse because you're just stagnant.'

"I didn't understand it either at first. I tried to get him to stay home at the beginning of the summer, but every time

I'd say I guessed I didn't feel like partying, he'd just call Mike or somebody else. I'd never seen him like that before.

"I remember one night, going to the Whalers' Club. He was trying to walk — oh, hell, it was only a block — and he kept clutching his side, and he had to stop three or four times, but he wouldn't let me help him. He was sweating all over, and his chest kept flapping in and out, and his eyes seemed to be asking, What's wrong with me?

"God, I was frightened, and I finally said something like, 'Sam, maybe if you rested up a couple of days, everything would be fine,' but he just shook his head and kept going. It didn't seem possible that he could get up and go to work the next day, but I knew he would."

Freddie had been absently rubbing the dog's back with his foot while he talked, but he stopped then and looked down as if he were surprised to find her there. He was obviously back on a warm summer night on Exchange Street with Sam.

"God, I was frightened," he said again, "and after that night Sam wouldn't even talk to me about it. I think he just decided then he was going to hang in there as long as he could, but I knew he was scared. It really depressed me, and all the other guys kept wondering why somebody didn't do something."

I was almost crying. "Oh, Fred," I interrupted, "don't think we didn't try. It's just we couldn't make him stop."

"I didn't mean that, Mrs. Poole," he said, so quickly that guilt couldn't even become an issue. "I mean that's when I began to understand what he was doing. He wanted to live so much, and being sick and just slowly dying wasn't living for him. Once the transplant thing came along and he knew he had something to fight for and a chance to really live again, he could psych himself up for it.

"Nobody else could understand how he could play it so cool about going out there. They thought a doctor or somebody had worked on him, but I knew it wasn't that. It was just Sam. Once he knows what he wants to do, nothing can make him give it up."

If I gotta, I gotta. I can handle it.

I could hear Sam saying it, back at Stanford, but before I could pull myself together to thank Freddie and tell him I thought I understood, he said, "I talked to Sam on the phone the other day, and he told me if he'd ever looked at the whole thing from an intellectual standpoint, he'd never have made it. It would have frightened him too much. He says he never asked 'Why me?' then, and he doesn't now."

His foot was back rubbing the dog's back, and suddenly he started to chuckle.

"You know what Sam told me, Mrs. Poole? He said, 'I just wake up in the morning, Fred, and ask myself what I can do to get better quicker and get the hell home, and then I do it. No big deal!' " Freddie smiled at me. "Maybe you oughta look at it that way too, Mrs. Poole," he said. "No big deal."

Moriah gave a massive yawn at that, and we both laughed, and Freddie looked down at his watch.

"I gotta go," he said. "I gotta meet my father in town," and he stood up, but instead of rushing off he fished a cigarette out of his shirt pocket, and a diabolical grin spread slowly over his face.

"Sam told me Dr. Hall dropped in on him too," he said.

I had finished the ironing, and I dropped my efforts in the laundry basket with a groan. "Oh, no, Freddie! And I suppose he told you what his father said to Dr. Hall too." Looking at Freddie's face, I could see there was no doubt that Sam had.

Dr. Hall, the cardiologist who had told us a heart transplant was years down the road for Sam, had evidently gone to San Francisco for a medical meeting. While tact had never been his strong point (I could still hear him saying right in front of Sam, "It would be easier for him if he had more intellectual interests, wouldn't it?"), he outdid himself when he appeared masked, gowned, and unannounced at Sam's door. It was his first error, for no outsider is ever supposed to visit a transplant room without the consent of the occupant.

"I bet you don't know who I am," he said.

That was his second mistake and a foolhardy game to play with Parker, who hates to be taken unaware.

"I don't know what came over. me," Parker reported, "but there was Sam, sitting up in bed, alive, and I thought where he'd be if we'd listened to Dr. Hall, and I heard myself saying, "That was *some* acid indigestion Sam had, wasn't it, doctor?'

"And, you know," Parker finished shamelessly, "it felt damned good saying it. I know it was nice of him to come all the way down from San Francisco to see Sam, but who the hell does he think he is, playing guessing games? That's no way to come into a room."

"I thought it was great," Fred exclaimed with enthusiasm. "God, Sam said all along the guy treated him as if he were totally ignorant, and that can't help when you're sick."

I had forgotten that, but it was just what Sam had written in his journal, after he'd learned about the transplant. I could see the words as plainly as if they were in front of me: "I'm sure I was ignorant to him, but I'm still human, and explaining things and saying why should be a big part of being sick. I think he thought I wasn't capable of handling the truth."

I repeated the words, and Freddie started to laugh. "Well, he didn't know Sam very well, did he? He's capable of handling anything. He just did!" He leaned down and gave me a kiss. "I really miss him, Mrs. Poole — all the guys do — it's pretty quiet around here without him. I can't wait till he gets home. My phone bill can't either," he finished dismally. "Are you going out there when Mr. Poole gets back?"

"Not for another week," I said. "Aunt Roz is taking the duty so Mr. Poole and I can do the income tax."

I hate income-tax time. It is Parker's annual dark night of the soul, and his mood blackens daily as April 15 approaches, but I was startled to find that this year a total eclipse was already in effect when he came back from California, and it was only March 21.

Parker's premature bleakness of spirit had been precipitated by the arrival in Palo Alto of Parker Poole III. Carried away by his new godson's birthday coinciding with that of his favorite saint, Pokie had heartily toasted both all the way from Portland to San Francisco, including a long stopover en route in Boston. He had arrived at the plastic apartment in no condition to bring cheer and comfort to the sick and had collapsed in a heap on the sofa.

"Goddammit, Pokie," Parker had roared at him, "I watched Sam dying on that sofa for two months. I'm not going to watch you. Get the hell up and go to bed." Three days after the fact and back in Portland, he was still fuming about it.

He fumed about everything all that week. It was the first time we'd been home together in almost four months, and I rapidly began to think I wouldn't care if it was the last. The money we'd saved for taxes had been used up long since on our new bicoastal living arrangements, the bills for the house were still coming in, and we were becoming far too intimate with the bank's loan officers. To add to the gloom, Parker said he'd found out the day he came home that Sam would definitely have to have a permanent pacemaker put in, and because of that he couldn't move to self-care.

"They want to keep him in ICU until they get it installed and are sure it's running properly," he told me. "I don't think staying there bothers him a bit — he says he'd miss his nurses — but I know the pacemaker does. He'd accepted being dependent on the medicines before he even got the heart, but needing a machine to stay alive surprised him. It bothers his vanity too, I think. He's afraid it's going to show."

The only thing that was entirely to Parker's liking was the new apartment. It would be ready and waiting for me on April 1, since everyone thought that Sam would be able to leave the hospital — pacemaker and all — by April 2 or 3.

"Moving from the plastic apartment will be a breeze for you, Vic," Parker said. "After all, what have you got to move?"

I didn't say a word, and I tried to be obliging all week. I cosigned the income tax, I cosigned the bank loans, but I was far from jubilant on the plane heading west, and the letter I'd gotten from Tina saying, "I told you not to worry, Mum. He says he isn't an ax murderer," created dismal food for thought.

"I just hope he doesn't dump you off in a fit of pique somewhere between Scylla and Charybdis," I wrote her back gloomily that day on the plane, care of American

Express in Athens, but I felt as if I were between them myself.

I was worried about moving. I'd barely had time to feed and care for myself on my last tour of duty with Sam, and I couldn't imagine where, regardless of what Parker said, I was going to find the hours to dismantle, clean, and vacate the plastic. I was even more worried about the pacemaker. I had no idea when it was going to be put in, but I knew it required surgery to do it, and the phone lines at the Cape had been out of order for three days because of an ice storm. I hadn't talked to Sam or Rozzie since.

This just won't do, I scolded myself; you can't go out there this ugly. And I finally managed to cheer up, remembering the phone calls I'd had from them before the storm. The aunt and the nephew were always in bad company when they were together, and bad company suited their tastes to perfection.

They had both been outraged the first time they'd called. A friend of Sam's from Kent had come to visit him, and, instead of agreeing as everyone else did that the transplant looked just like Jesus, he had said, "Well, no offense, but Charles Manson's more like it, if you ask me."

With the next call they were ecstatic. Rozzie had spotted a bulge in Sam's arm she was convinced was muscle, when he was lifting weights in physical therapy.

Their last call before the phones went out was the one I liked the best, though. Rozzie had been complaining that Sam was turning his daily walks outside into Olympic training sessions. "Every day it's longer, and farther, and faster, and me with high heels," she'd groan, but this particular day, when they'd already walked for a good half hour, he decided he wanted to explore the area behind the graduate schools. Kathy was with them, and when she

heard that she said it was her lunchtime and it would be a
great chance for Sam to be on his own for the first time.

"I'll meet you back at the hospital in an hour," she said.
"It'll take you that long anyway. The graduate schools are
to hell and gone from here," and she departed, abandoning
the patient and Rozzie.

"Oh, it was awful, Aunt Vic," she'd wailed to me over the
phone. "I felt as if I'd been handed the controls of a seven-
forty-seven jet. All I could think of was Sam falling down,
or going into cardiac arrest, or rejecting, and I didn't even
know where we were going, and he wouldn't wait for me,
and I had to gallop just to keep him in range."

It didn't take much imagination to see the scene. Sam
had adopted the procession as his mode of travel as soon as
he was let out of his room. He said no man could be expected to listen to woman talk all day, and I could just see
Rozzie, as I had often done myself, running breathlessly
after his swiftly advancing booties.

It took even less to picture her consternation when, walking through a secluded woods, he stopped and called back
to her, "Hey, Aunt Roz, did you see that gorilla on the
leash?"

"I knew it had to be the drugs he was taking," Rozzie
said, "so while he was stopped, looking off into the trees, I
caught up with him and took hold of his arm. I was very
firm. 'No, Sam,' I said, 'I did not see a gorilla on a leash.
Come along. We have walked a long way now, and we
should go back to Kathy.' "

But Sam just stared at her, she said, as if *she* were the
one who was hallucinating, and while she wondered with
mounting panic what she would do if he refused to come
with her, he started to laugh. "Look, Aunt Roz," he had finally sputtered out. "Look over there."

She did, and, as she described it: "There, gamboling through the eucalyptus, O blessed sight — out with his keeper, just like Sam, for an afternoon stroll — was a real, great big, hairy, dear old gorilla. I could have kissed him!"

It turned out to be the gorilla that Stanford is teaching to talk, and I was very grateful to him all the way to San Francisco. I couldn't have felt cheerier when Rozzie picked me up at the airport at seven o'clock, and by the time I got into bed that night, I had also felt startled, bewildered, and ecstatic.

What startled me was Sam. He was having the pacemaker put in at the very moment Rozzie picked me up, and, driving down to the hospital, she had handled the car as if she were in the Grand Prix. It had been an awful three days, she said, and she'd tell me about it later, but right now she wanted to get back to the hospital so we'd be there when Sam got back to his room.

He wasn't there, and we paced nervously up and down in the hall, waiting. Rozzie's mind was obviously on nothing but Sam's return.

"What is it? Is it something awful?" I asked her once or twice, but she only shook her head and said "Later" and continued her pacing. When a stretcher finally did appear, surrounded by three of Sam's nurses, I was prepared for the worst — certainly not for the noisy protests that were coming from the stretcher's occupant.

"God, I'm starved! These damn operations are screwing up my whole digestive track."

I breathed a sigh of relief. However awful the last three days had been, Sam sounded quite like himself, but when I bent over the stretcher to kiss him hello he didn't look like himself at all. I could have been kissing a complete stranger. It wasn't just the new masses of beard either. In the three weeks I'd been gone, the shape of his face had totally changed. Above his mask and below his bonnet swelled the rounded puffy cheeks of the prednisone-taker. Even the beard, bristling fiercely around the mask, couldn't hide them, and I remember thinking for one miserable second, He's not Sam anymore; but he said "Hi, Mum" with such delight in his voice that I forgot all about his looks in my own delight at being with him again.

Sam's looks surely didn't seem to bother him, nor did the pacemaker. His stomach seemed to be his only concern, and it was only after Judy produced the dietetic chocolate-cream pie she'd made for him, and he'd contentedly rubbed his stomach and said, "I can't believe I ate the whole thing," that he even mentioned his newest operation.

Then he did ask us a couple of times, "Do you think it shows an awful lot?" and he did twist his head awkwardly once or twice to peer at it, and admittedly it did show. It looked as if someone had somehow slipped a Zippo lighter just under the skin next to his left shoulder, below the collarbone, but once his nurses assured him that, the way he built up muscle, no one would know it was there in a month, he ignored it altogether.

Rozzie had seemed to relax the minute Sam came back, but she hardly spoke going home to the apartment. I was completely bewildered until she collapsed on the gilt-flecked plastic of one of the dining-room chairs, put her head down on the table, and said, "Make me a drink, please. I feel as if I'd just spent a whole week with Daddy!"

The week had evidently begun with selecting the pacemaker. Sam wanted to know exactly what model was going to be put inside him and exactly how it would look.

"You'd have thought it was you and me going over the Bergdorf catalog the way he and Dr. Baumgartner went over the available types and varieties," Rozzie said, and after Dr. B left the room, Sam spent hours weighing the merits of that day's possibilities, judging each by two firm guidelines: the pacemaker mustn't show, and it mustn't move when he did. "After they finally picked one," she said, "he never brought the subject up again."

Then they'd concentrated on getting the pacemaker operation scheduled. Rozzie said that Sam had been great about it. He had been supposed to have it installed the day before I came out, but the operating rooms had been too busy. Sam's operation had been scratched at six o'clock that night, after he had fasted all day. At midnight he'd had to start in fasting all over again.

"He never complained once," Rozzie said, "but this morning they told him he'd probably have to have ATG shots for a while after he left the hospital, and, what with the pacemaker mess, it just seemed like the last straw. I think he thought once he got to the new apartment the worst would be behind him. He kept saying over and over, 'They never told me that before. Nobody ever told me that,' and he looked so sunk I couldn't bear it."

"Well, he certainly wasn't sunk tonight," I said, feeling that Rozzie was getting a little melodramatic. I reached around behind my chair to retrieve my cigarettes from the kitchen. "He was on the crest of the wave. God, Rozzie, you look a hell of a lot more as though you'd had an operation than he does."

"You're not listening again," she stated in the aggravated tones often employed by older sisters. "Didn't I just tell you I felt as if I'd spent a week with Daddy? Have you forgotten how *he* used to act when something he didn't expect came along? He'd think about it, he'd talk about it, he'd go over it and over it until you thought you'd go mad, but once he'd decided how he was going to cope with it, he'd never bother to tell you. The next night, when you'd ask him how things were going with whatever it was, he'd bang on the desk and say, 'Goddammit, what the hell are you beating that dead horse for?' as if you'd been the one doing all the talking."

She paused and took one of my cigarettes.

"I," she said pointedly, "haven't had time to buy cigarettes this week," and then she laughed. "At least Sam never started goddamming at me, but the minute I saw him tonight after the operation, I knew he'd accepted the ATG the same way he'd accepted the pacemaker once he realized he had to have it. It was just one more dead horse for him, exactly as it would have been for Daddy, and *I* was the one in the state of collapse. I tell you it's really shaken me up to be back playing dear old Dad's game after two years."

"I know," I said. "I've just learned the name of it. It's called 'If I gotta, I gotta.'"

They'd made plans for moving just as competently. Hearing how they'd done it produced my fourth mood of the day, ecstasy. Sam was going to have to be bedridden and reattached to the heart monitor for the next twenty-four hours to be sure that the pacemaker was pacing properly, but after that he was going to be transferred to self-care for a couple of days and would be able to move to the new apartment on April 3.

"You couldn't leave him all alone in the hospital while you moved," Rozzie said. "Who'd get him his popsicles?" and with that she announced that she was going to stay in California to help me and that Uncle Bill was coming out for the weekend to baby-sit with Sam while we worked.

"It was all Sam's idea," she said modestly, as I threw my arms around her.

There isn't a doubt in my mind to this day that if Rozzie hadn't stayed and Bill hadn't come, I would never have survived. First, we had to transfer Sam and his mounds of belongings out of ICU into self-care. It seemed wasted energy to me at the beginning. I couldn't see how two days without his nurses were going to make him fit to face the outside world, but it seemed that a stint in self-care, however brief, was a must on the road to recovery. No transplant could leave the hospital for good until experimental passes out had been made, and only transplants in self-care were allowed to make them.

"That seems silly," I'd said to Kathy, who'd responded, "Not half as silly as you'd seem, moving into your new apartment with Sam in his bonnet and booties. Don't forget, all transplants in ICU have to be gowned up to leave their rooms." I leapt into packing him up with a will after that.

In truth, Rozzie did most of the work of moving Sam while I went to the airport to pick up Bill. When we got back to the hospital, I didn't even recognize the tall, thin, bearded young man who strode down the hall toward us. Only the blue mask he wore suggested that he might possibly be a patient. It wasn't till I identified the cutoff painting shorts and the tattered red rowing shirt and saw the untied Adidas that I realized it was Sam. He was dressed in his own clothes for the first time in two months, and when he saw Bill the stride almost became a run.

"Hi, Uncle Bill," he roared with delight.

Embracing him, Uncle Bill exclaimed, "My boy, you're my first miracle. God heard my call."

317

"It's a good thing he didn't hear what you called him, Uncle Bill," Sam said, and Rozzie and I abandoned the care and feeding of our heart transplant to our new assistant.

Swinging into the full gear that had enabled us together to dismantle three huge houses in as many months, we confronted the plastic. It was, however, almost more of a challenge. I snarled Parker's "After all, what have you got to move?" at every drawer, bulging with get-well cards, and every closet, heaped with the presents Sam had been too sick to look at when he lived there and now said he wanted. At least at home there had been boxes, and rubbish men, and suitcases, and, although we did have a moving man, when the time came to move, Bill couldn't concentrate on being useful. The results of the ATG shots had finished him.

Sam was only having ATG every three or four days by that time, and his legs had looked almost normal. Bill watched Sam have the shots the first night he came quite unperturbed, but the next noon, after he had deposited Sam in the new apartment for his first pass out of the hospital, he appeared at the plastic in genuine shock.

"Sam got into bed the minute we got there," he said. "The poor kid can hardly walk. His knees are all swollen, and it looks as if someone has pounded his legs with a sledgehammer. You wouldn't believe it!"

Rozzie and I were unsympathetically blasé. "Oh, yes, we would," we said. "Now help us carry this stuff down to the car."

What I wouldn't have believed was my sadness at leaving. California's curtain-cleaning law seemed to have been forgotten, and new tenants were lugging in their suitcases as Rozzie and I lugged ours out. "You haven't even had a chance to see if I left it clean," I protested to the landlady. Her reply — "Oh, don't worry about that; I saw the way you kept it when I showed the new people around" — filled me with proprietary pride, and before I threw the last bag into the car, I stood for a second and looked up at our balcony and my watchcat's balcony below it. "Good-bye, little cabin," I said out loud, Rozzie squeezed my hand, and unbelievably, tears ran down my cheeks all the way to the new apartment.

Before Parker came home he had toured it with its owner, and I knew just where it was because it was clearly visible from the hospital. It was part of a huge complex called Oak Creek, and, as Uncle Bill drove us up to our new estate, I couldn't not be impressed. At least fifteen separate buildings stretched across manicured velvet lawns. Vines, flowers, trees, and shrubs surrounded each building.

Uncle Bill said, "It's interesting to see how the California drought stops right at the edge of the Oak Creek property." Viewing the unaccustomed lushness, I remember feeling as if the occupants of Ma's Boarding House had moved to the Ritz.

With Uncle Bill's help, Aunt Roz and I, in our dungarees, dragged our belongings into the exotic smoked-glass-and-chrome decor of the building's entryway. The orange plastic dishpan laden with cleaning supplies, the torn paper bags, and the crumbling cartons we had salvaged from the refuse heap behind the plastic apartment looked depressingly déclassé.

"Think Louis Vuitton," Rozzie said calmly, as we loaded up the elevator under the baleful eye of an immaculately dressed-for-tennis tenant.

It wasn't easy. I still felt like a burglar as Uncle Bill unlocked the door of our apartment on the second floor and ushered us in. Picasso and Matisse prints decorated three of the art-gallery-beige walls of the living room; the fourth was glass and opened onto a grassy terrace edged with trees and shrubs.

"Walk gently when you go outside," Uncle Bill warned. "I figured out that the terrace is built on top of your car down in the garage."

I simply couldn't believe my eyes. "Look, Rozzie," I kept exclaiming as I led her past a movie-set built-in bar to the left of the living room, past a marvelously unplastic dining-room table, and into the kitchen. Everything we'd been lacking before was spread before us, but after I'd led her back through the living room for a tour to the right — of a well-stocked linen closet, two bathrooms, and two bedrooms — she shook her head sadly.

"I ought to feel like Sarah Crewe," she said, "but I don't. I think I'm going to be homesick. I understood the plastic."

If Uncle Bill had been shattered by Sam's legs, he was awed by his next foray into the world of heart transplanting. It took place the night we moved. Leaving Rozzie to wash the dishes, he and I had driven Sam, feverish from the shots and exhausted by his first pass, back to the hospital. All the other transplants had left Stanford by then, and I remember saying to Sam as we got out of the car, "Dr. Shumway's got to get busy. When you leave, day after tomorrow, he won't have any transplants to play with at all."

Dr. Shumway was way ahead of me. No sooner had Sam gotten into bed than a knock came at his door and a tall man, quite handsome, but gray beneath his tan, came slowly into the room. He was dressed in white hospital pajamas and bathrobe, and he looked tired and miserable.

"I'm Jeff Ogilvey," he said to Sam, and his voice sounded

as tired and miserable as he looked. "They told me you wouldn't mind if I came and talked to you. I'm having a heart transplant tomorrow, and I just hate the thought of it. Is it terrible?"

He must have been twenty years older than Sam, but there was genuine fear in his voice, and I couldn't imagine how, knowing how awful Sam felt himself that night, he could possibly pull himself together enough to be encouraging. I turned my head toward him anxiously, but there wasn't a trace left of the tired, feverish eighteen-year-old boy. Sitting up and leaning forward eagerly to talk to Jeff, he was giving more than compassion. He was giving himself.

"Gee, don't be afraid, Jeff," he said. "You've already gotten through the worst. When you're waiting, and nothing's happening, and you just hurt all over, that's the bad time. After tomorrow it won't hurt you to breathe anymore, and, oh, God, it's so great just to live again."

"But you don't understand," Jeff Ogilvey said, and his voice was now protesting. "I've had cardiomyopathy for seven years, and it's never bothered me the way the thought of tomorrow does. I understood that I'd have time to get used to the idea of having a transplant while I waited for a heart. I only got accepted into the program yesterday, and I haven't had any time to wait at all. I don't think it's fair for them to spring it on me like this."

Nothing Sam could say seemed to reach him at all. He watched quietly as the man left his room, and after the door closed he shook his head.

"He won't be able to handle it," he said to Uncle Bill and me. "It's not his fault, but he'll never make it if he doesn't want it. You've got to want to live more than anything else in the world. You've got to want to live so much that nothing else can bother you no matter how long you wait, or how much it hurts, or anything else."

Bill didn't say a word all the way back to Oak Creek, and once we got to the apartment he went out on the terrace and sat for a long time. I was in the living room talking to Rozzie, and when he finally came back in he said, "How old is Sam?" and — after I told him — "That's not what I was thinking about when I was eighteen," and went to bed.

I couldn't sleep that night. I could hear Freddie saying, "He wanted to live so much, and being sick and just slowly dying wasn't living for him," and finally I knew that the very thing that had made Sam live might kill Jeff Ogilvey. Sam had refused to accept being sick.

Bill went with me again to pick him up for good on April 3 at nine o'clock in the morning. It was precisely four months to the day since Sam's eighteenth birthday and his acceptance into the heart transplant program. It was precisely two months to the day since his new birthday, and Uncle Bill insisted on recording the occasion with his camera. There for posterity stand Sam and I foolishly waving good-bye to the braying doors of Stanford Medical Center, but it wasn't until the picture was developed that I realized the significance of what I was wearing that morning. Without even thinking I had put on the same pristine white pants and white T-shirt with pink teardrops spattered on it that I'd worn the horrible day, almost a year ago, when Dr. Wakely had told us Sam was going to die.

Nobody was thinking about dying that morning or was even depressed by lugging into the lobby at Oak Creek the bewildering array of boxes and bags filled with the paraphernalia from which a heart transplant should not be separated: his pills and his potions, his masks and his pill cups.

"By damn, Sam," I said, as Bill pushed the button for the elevator, "if you don't watch out, you're going to get to the top of that glass mountain, and you'll have to end up marrying the princess."

"Not me," he said. "Catch 'em young, treat 'em rough, and tell 'em nothing — that's my motto," and he had to be forcibly reminded by his mother that ladies enter elevators first.

A friend at home had sent out a huge box mysteriously labeled SAM'S INSTANT COMING-OUT PARTY, and Uncle Bill had opened it that morning before we went to the hospital. It was filled with paper hats, horns, leis, a huge cardboard Maine lobster, and an even bigger paper banner with *Welcome Home, Sam* written on it. Ignoring the puzzled glances of the four apartment dwellers who shared the second-floor terrace with us, Bill had set up the party outside, and as Sam walked out through the sliding glass doors of the living room, a champagne cork popped by Uncle Bill saluted the long-awaited return of Transplant 120 to the outside world.

It was not the only cork to be popped that day. Before my return, Lynn had left for a three-week trip to Hawaii to be married, but Judy and Kathy came to visit their ex-patient. After Sam put on his "I Left My Heart in San Francisco" T-shirt, and amidst the din of the paper horns and the toasts, I began to wonder if we'd be evicted by nightfall.

The neighbors didn't bother Uncle Bill a bit. "Come meet my nephew," he invited an elderly gentleman who was trying to read his newspaper in the sun. "You've got a celebrity living next door to you," and the man, who said his name was Ed, obligingly got up and shook Sam's hand while Rozzie and the nurses and I dove back into the apartment in mortification.

When Rozzie finally shrieked, "My God, it's seven thirty and we haven't even packed up to go home, Bill Richardson — we'll miss our plane!" I couldn't imagine where the day had gone.

Uncle Bill didn't seem to be contemplating a trip back to Maine at all, and only at the zero hour did he wobble out of the building with his Philadelphia hat askew.

Rozzie and I were waiting for him in the car. "Do you think he'll be mad if I drive?" I whispered nervously to her.

"Don't bother to ask him," she said. "Just drive," and we departed for the airport with Uncle Billy protesting noisily that he wasn't ready to go home at all, he liked California, and he loved nurses.

When I got back from the airport, I discovered that the heart transplant had washed all the dishes — and *that* was enough excitement for one day.

Chapter Thirteen

If I had more than one batch of clean dishes to produce as testimony to the success of Stanford's heart transplant program, I'd write "And so they all lived happily ever after" and go back to washing my woodwork. But unfortunately those dishes are the only ones I remember Sam doing the entire time we were at Oak Creek. There weren't enough hours in his day to waste on dishes. It was a full-time occupation just becoming plain old Sam again — or rather, as he had written over his pajama hook in the bathroom at the cottage when he was seven: TALCOTT SIMES POOLE, THE GREAT.

Oak Creek was a perfect place for him to do his becoming in. It had a gymnasium, a massage room, a sauna, and a steam bath. It had tennis courts (only one paddle-tennis court — but after all . . .), an Olympic-sized swimming pool, and even a Jacuzzi.

Personally, it was not my cup of tea. It was a lovely place, but it bothered me. There wasn't a cat or a dog to be seen, and children were in evidence only between the hours of twelve and one. The swimming-pool rules stated firmly that no one under fifteen was allowed in it except at those hours, and in fact the only annoyance the tanned inhabitants of Oak Creek seemed unable to contend with was the temperature of the pool. Let it fall below 80 degrees, as it did upon occasion, and it was as if the Four Horsemen of the Apocalypse were charging roughshod through the wisteria-covered pool gates. To someone accustomed to Maine water and conditioned to a more eclectic population, life at Oak Creek rapidly began to assume a dreamlike two-dimensional quality. Only when one of Sam's nurses (or a friend from Kent or home) came to visit did I feel really awake and alive. Fortunately they came with great regularity, and despite my misgivings about our environment, even I, particularly at the beginning, wouldn't have wanted to be any farther away from the hospital than we were.

Contemplating Sam in his civvies, I had no question as to the wisdom of Stanford's philosophy that transplants must stay in the area for a while. Regardless of Rozzie's sighting of a muscle bulge, no one six-foot-two-inches tall who weighs 126 pounds looks in the pink. "Frail" is the only possible word to describe Sam as we settled down together to our new mode of living.

Uncle Bill had announced on the day of the coming-out party that "the boy needs muscling up" and had taken him to the pool for his first swim. Rozzie and I had passed them, as we set off for a walk twenty minutes later. They were both still dry, sitting in chairs at the edge of the pool. Sam was staring at it, and Uncle Bill, flourishing a large cigar, was obviously encouraging him to give it a try.

We came back a good half hour later, and they were still sitting and still dry. It seemed like ages before they reappeared at the apartment, and although they were both wet, Bill was obviously distressed.

When Sam went into his room to change clothes, Bill took me into the kitchen. "He's in terrible shape," he said. "I didn't think he was going to make one lap up the pool, even though he made himself do five, but it took forever. My God, he's like an old man of eighty. You'll have to keep an eye on him. He had to lie down on a pool chair after he got out of the water."

Looking at his medicines jamming the medicine cabinet, tumbling off the shelves, swarming over his bureau, piled in his closet, I liked Stanford's stay-close policy even better. The drugs were still terrifying unknown quantities to me, although they didn't seem to confuse Sam a bit; and, scouring his shower and his sink in my daily war against germs, I was relieved that the hospital was only three minutes away and that Sam had to report to clinic, as all released transplants did, twice a week.

Three minutes away too — and the salvation of my days — was the Stanford dietitian. No one who has avoided cooking like the plague for almost half a century and who is asked by Dottie, after every day off, "Well, what did you burn for dinner last night?" could leap with joy into cooking for a heart transplant. No salt, no sugar, no cholesterol — the three nos seemed to be in everything I knew how to cook, and prepared foods of any sort were strictly off the list; they all had salt in them. Putting a lifetime of Campbell's soup behind me, I turned to the dietitian. She managed to drill into me some menus I could cope with and Sam didn't seem to mind, but we ate salads till I could feel the alfalfa sprouts clustering in my ears.

Like the ad "Leave the driving to us," it was great to leave the important worrying to Stanford, but it put me in a rather tenuous position. I didn't know what role to play, although Sam seemed to know instantly the ones I shouldn't. Looking back I think he was absolutely right, but I did a lot of tongue-biting the first few days. Once I realized that everything he did was to speed his recovery and, as he had said to Fred, "to get the hell home," I relaxed a little.

From morning till night, allowing for the fact that only on clinic days did he get up at anything that could decently be called morning, he worked to make himself well. And if it was Sam's kingdom we were living in, he was a very benevolent despot and I, his solitary subject, rarely rebellious.

I learned that I was not to be a protective mother as soon as I got back from taking Bill and Rozzie to the airport.

"Leave the car keys on the table when you go to bed, will ya?" he yelled at me from his room. "I gotta be at clinic at seven o'clock in the morning."

And to my "Oh, dear Lord, Sam, you haven't driven since November. Do you think you'll remember how?" through the door came a disgusted "Gawd, Mum," and I put the keys on the table.

I got up, of course, to hover over his departure. "How do you feel?" I asked.

It was a strictly routine question. Since he'd gotten his heart, it was such a joy to hear him say "Fine" that I asked it, I know, much too regularly. He was quite justified in saying pleasantly but very firmly that first morning, "I feel fine. How do you feel? You worry about how you feel; I'll worry about me."

I was not, I decided, to be a nervous mother either. That decision was reinforced when he came back from clinic. He told me his precise medical condition: his voltage was the same, he'd put on two pounds — they thought from yesterday's celebrating — but when I asked what we ought to do about it, he said, "Not we, Mum. Me," and I subsided while he brought me up to date on the progress of the other transplants he'd seen there.

His independent noninvalid status established as the first step toward "getting the hell home," he turned immediately to the second, his body. He worked out in the gym that same morning, and when he came back he made a very involved chart, recording fifteen leg lifts, twelve chest pulls, and innumerable other feats of strength that meant nothing to me. By nightfall he had added to the chart not the ten laps in the pool I'd heard him promise Uncle Bill he'd try for, but fourteen.

From a remote chair, hidden behind a wisteria vine so no one could possibly presume me to be a relative, I had watched him. It had taken him a long time. At the end his arms were flailing wildly, not stroking, but when I watched him pull himself out over the edge of the pool — disdaining the steps — I felt the same joy I'd felt when Charlie's Kent boat was first to cross the finish line at Henley.

After the swim was even better. On two long chairs in the sun lay Sam and a friend from Kent who'd dropped in. I could see Sam's scar and the bulge where his pacemaker was because I knew they were there, but I don't think they were noticed by the girls that he and Andy were ogling from behind their shades.

"Laid back, catching the rays," I murmured to myself, feeling very Californian.

I was so ecstatic at seeing him on his own, in a world not peopled by parents and doctors and nurses, that I agreed without thinking to the role he finally did select for me that night. I was to be his tennis partner, beginning the very next day. Right then I would have vastly preferred to be allowed to be a protective mother, or a nervous mother, or

both. Swimming was one thing, but tearing around an asphalt tennis court was another, and I was feeling very edgy
as we set off.

We climbed down the ladder that was a shortcut from
our terrace to the pool and the courts, and Sam signed up
for a court; I suggested that we go to the one farthest away
from the onlookers and the pro who was giving a lesson.

Despite the plumpness of Sam's cheeks, to the spectators
it must have looked as if someone had girded up the loins
and thrust a tennis racket into the right hand of a Christ
risen from the dead. A sea of eyes were upon us as we
crossed the courts.

It goes without saying that, being me, I hit the first shot
wide of Sam's reach, and it also goes without saying that,
with his legs still swollen and stiff from the ATG and
weak from disuse, he crashed down onto the asphalt.

There were gasps from the other courts. I wanted to rush
over to the other side to help him up, but I knew it would in-
furiate him, so instead I stood on my own side, toying
with my racket as casually as though he were well padded
and not a bleeder.

Out of the corner of my eye, I could see the neighbor to
whom Uncle Bill had introduced Heart Transplant 120
whispering to the other spectators. Finally and agoniz-
ingly Sam got up, avoiding his knees in a sort of roll-
around sit-up. His leg was bleeding.

"Okay?" I called.

"Yeah," he said, "sorry," and he hit a ball to me.

Despite his medicines he wasn't bleeding too badly, and
the Lord must have directed my shots into his proper
range because I never could have on my own. We played for
more than half an hour, and it was I who called it quits.

330

I couldn't stand another minute of wondering if the blood was going to clot properly.

"That's enough for the mother," I announced. "You're about to give me emphysema." And without argument we started back toward the apartment.

Halfway back I realized that I'd left my sweater on the court, and returning to retrieve it I ran into the neighbor.

"I saw what happened," he said. "I can't believe a heart transplant should be playing tennis."

"Oh, exercise is the best thing," I said cheerily, but I had a horrible feeling inside that if Dr. Shumway had witnessed Sam's fall he would have agreed with our neighbor.

I picked up my sweater with my head down, hoping, ostrichlike, not to be further noticed, but the pro was just leaving his court. "I watched your son," he said. "He's got good strokes, and I think I could help him a lot with those bum legs of his. Tell him the pro is an old guy who knows all kinds of tricks to get around a court without having to run."

I could have kissed him. For the first time that day, I didn't feel like an irresponsible mother.

The hospital wasn't at all excited about Sam's leg. They told him casually not to fall down anymore, and all I was left to be concerned about were my transplant patient's mask habits. He would not wear one, as I understood he should. He shoved one in his pocket when he went to clinic and said he put it on when he got there, but he wouldn't take one to San Francisco the day we went, and when he went off to Santa Cruz with five friends from Maine for a party there, he bit my head off when I suggested that he take one along.

It was so great to see him swing out the door, laughing

and saying, "See ya, Mum, I'll be back sometime," that I didn't insist, but all night I felt I should have.

The next day when Judy came for lunch, I said — right in front of Sam so he'd hear her answer — "Judy, Sam doesn't wear a mask anywhere except to the hospital. Tell him he has to."

The black hair was unbraided that day. Judy's face was solemn, and she pushed back her hair and thought for a minute before she answered.

"You don't, Sam?" she said with such shocked disapproval that I was sure she would uphold me — until I saw the eyes crinkle and heard the giggle; I was going to be shot down, I knew — and I was.

"That's what we always tell transplants at the beginning. If they know the very worst that can happen beforehand, it's not such a blow afterward. If you'd been very susceptible to infection, Sam, you would have to wear a mask in public. We'd have made a big thing out of it, and rather than catch something you probably wouldn't have minded too much. After all, we'd told you you were going to have to wear one all along. You're just lucky. There are a lot of things you may be able to do that you thought you couldn't, and things you don't have to do that you thought you would."

"Like what?" Sam asked eagerly, but Judy's face had gone back to being inscrutable.

"Like not having to put up with ATG after you got out of the hospital. And there'll be others," she said enigmatically, and while she cautioned again that under no circumstances must he ever go into a hospital without a mask ("That's where all the germs are"), it was a relief not to have to worry about face coverings and him and the public bars anymore.

Instead I turned my attentions to my own moral fiber and found it in sad disarray. I was swimming all day, lolling in the sun, and sitting in the sulphured waters of the Jacuzzi like a native. My Protestant work ethic was outraged.

"Wicked, wicked," I would mutter, finding myself, the day's chores completed, en route to the pool at nine thirty in the morning, and the letters from home only made me feel guiltier. I'd look out on the terrace at a neighbor who stood for hours every day doing what the lady next door said was Tai Chee and think, I want to go home. It couldn't be right, I knew, for a grown man to stand there, with a stupid self-loving expression on his face, doing what to my mind were damned weird things with his body.

"He oughta get a job," I grumbled morosely to myself one morning, stomping away from the glass doors where I'd been watching. Thankfully I didn't read Ruthie's letter till the man had finished doing his thing for the day or I might have yelled it out loud.

Her letter started off with news about Tina's arrival at home. "She looks *fantastic*," Ruthie wrote, "and her room is a shambles so you *know* she's home," and then she flatteringly said, "I need my mother-in-law to coach me with this damn kid. Dottie gave me the word that you said to 'throw out the goddamned baby books,' and she made him stop crying the other day by saying firmly, 'Shut up, baby. I'm talking,' so I guess if you get home, between the two of you he'll end up O.K."

The end was the hardest to read. It described Parker's fiftieth birthday: "It was a great B-day party with toastings and asparagus with 'Holiday Sauce,' as Dottie calls it, lots of laughs, and good cheer in the new living room, which really looked lived in with Aunt Roz and Uncle Bill's new puppy making magic circles on the rug, Aunt Roz wiping them up, your own dear dog barking, little Gussie wailing, Uncle Billy laughing, Tina being Grecian, Pokie teasing Alix, and Uncle Parker spreading wrapping paper all over the floor — if only everyone could have been there, but we all said over and over again, *'It won't be long now!!!!'* "

I wanted to cry, but all I said was "Here" and handed Sam the letter.

We had a very quiet supper. Sam collapsed on the sofa watching TV, and I went into the kitchen to wash the dishes.

"Mum," I heard him say when I was almost finished, "do you think we could move back to the cottage this summer? I've never lived in the new house except when I was sick, and it would be kinda nice to be with Charlie again in the back room at the cottage feeling good," and I rushed in from the kitchen crying, "Oh, yes."

It wasn't till I woke up the next morning that I remembered that I had solemnly promised Parker and Dottie and all the children that, once we moved to the new house, I'd never make anybody move anywhere again.

The older children say Parker and I spoil Alix. We take her on exotic spring-vacation trips that they say will be her ruination, but which we say she deserves.

"She has to put up with the rest of you," we say to them, and then we tell Alix she's a spoiled only child, but nobody had given any thought to her spring vacation while Sam was sick until Tina came home.

With her clothes barely washed from the trip to Greece, she suggested that she bring Alix to California. I could take Al home after her vacation was over, and leave, as she put it, "the elderly ugly daughter in charge of the heart transplant for a while."

No sooner was that settled than a phone call came from Louise in Wyoming. "Aunt Vic," she said, "I'm out of the woods. Could you stand a very dirty niece for a week? I don't want to be the only Richardson not to see a miracle."

The thought of having all three of the family ladies to gossip with went to my head like champagne. I was sorely in need of reinforcements. I had sprained both ankles jogging by then and could barely hobble. Twenty daily laps in the pool, three sets of tennis and a tennis lesson, not to mention leg lifts and chest pulls, were turning Sam into his proper image of himself. His 140-pound weight, the hospital said, was pure muscle, and the entries on his exercise chart were staggering. His muscle bulges were inspirational, the pacemaker hardly showed, but his mother was a wreck.

With the arrival of the girls, the hushed silence of Oak Creek was shattered. To the courts, to the pool, to the gym strode the benevolent despot with his female army trailing behind. Sam had built up a coterie of admirers before they came, and I had seen people talking to him at the pool and asking him to play tennis at the courts, but I'd tried so hard not to be motherly that I didn't know any of them. The girls had no such inhibitions.

In the family, and with a certain amount of sarcasm, Tina's "Hi-I'm-Tina-Poole-from-Portland-Maine" is widely imitated. She hugs unknown babies, embraces the world, and there isn't an ounce of New England reserve in all six feet of her. She was a surprising and very visible addition to the poolside population of Oak Creek, and people who had never spoken to me before started nodding and smiling.

Louise added another dimension. Her slight build and little oval face, with its wide blue eyes and freckles, disguise the fact that she can scale mountains with hundred-pound packs on her back and never loses at anything. To keep herself in shape on her week off, she sprang up on any available doorway and effected ten or twelve quick chin-ups, which was obviously startling to the Tai Chee mentality of Oak Creek; and on the tennis court the pro was heard to say that she really didn't need a lesson. I soon was getting nods and smiles from the spectators there.

All this emboldened me to allow twelve-year-old Alix to swim from morning till night in a pool which specifically prohibited children under fifteen. Sam had said right at the beginning, "Aw, hell, tell her to act like she's fifteen. She does anyway," and I had — but guiltily. With our new social status courtesy of the children, and without a twinge, I was soon watching Alix, brown of hair and seallike of body, happily wallowing in the pool.

For the first time in four months, Sam was part of a visible family again. The only startling thing was that it was clear from the outset that the younger generation's pecking order had changed. For eighteen years Sam had stood sixth in order, as no two people knew better than Louise and Christina, who had devoted their childhood to making him aware of his lowly position.

No longer! They followed behind him as docilely as I had done before they came. Until we all went to San Francisco, though, I don't think either of them really understood why he would never be just a younger brother again. Louise was bored that day. Her heart was obviously still in the Wyoming highlands, and she had spent a good part of the morning breaking a cardinal rule of the Poole-Richardson households; in both, no one ever says "I don't care," but that morning it had been her exclusive answer to every "What shall we do now?" A tacky wax museum selected by Alix had evidently been the last straw for the intrepid wilderness leader, and she repaired to a bench on Fisherman's Wharf to stare silently and gloomily at Alcatraz and San Francisco Bay. Christina had abandoned ship without so much as a "by your leave" to buy sourdough bread, and I could see that Sam was annoyed.

In despair I took Alix across the street to buy a rug hooking set ("like his") she'd seen in a shop window, and, when I came back five minutes later, to my amazement, Louise was vibrant with enthusiasm, Christina was apologizing for her defection, and Sam was standing silent between them with a look of determined satisfaction.

When we were crossing the street to go to a restaurant, Louise fell back with me. "I'm sorry, Aunt Vic," she said. "I didn't mean to wreck Al's time." I knew she meant it. Louise does not dissemble.

"Forget it," I said. "It happens in the best families." But she hadn't finished.

"No," she said. "It was all the crowds, I guess. I'm not used to them, and I wasn't thinking of Alix at all. Sam let Tina and me have it. He said we weren't being fair to her."

She walked on a little way without speaking, and I knew she was weighing in her mind whether Sam had been absolutely justified in his attack. Being fair has been the sine qua non of Louise's life, but in a second or two she gave the little laugh that means she'll rise to fight another day and said, "It's funny. Sam was never like that before. I think if I were a heart transplant I'd be so busy worrying about me, I wouldn't have time to be fighting battles for Al or anyone else."

"Me neither," I said, and after that we had a ball, up to

and including waiting outside seven men's-rooms in seven San Franciscan hotels for Sam to pee.

I don't think Alix ever knew she had a champion. Sam kept his light well hidden under a bushel of brotherly abuse. The night the girls came he'd told her magnificently that she could sleep in the extra bed in his room. "But," he said, and he looked so pleased with himself as he handed her a Mycostatin lozenge that I couldn't prick his bubble, "not until you suck this. You have to be sanitary to sleep in my room."

Anxious to do the right thing, Alix put it in her mouth, and not until she was halfway through it did he say, "You know what you're eating, Al? It's a cure for VD," and the beige oval lozenge shot out damply onto the off-white shag of the living-room rug.

After that she ignored him and turned his supposedly sterile bathroom into what he complained was "a zit cream jungle." Whenever he went into it, angry mutterings could be heard through the door. "Chrissakes, the government's got millions in me. I oughta get a little respect."

Somewhere on the list of my failings, equaled only in length by my list of hers, Rozzie has put "single-mindedness." Although I'd never admit it to her, it's true. It wasn't till I got home with Al from California, leaving Sam hale and hearty at Oak Creek with Tina, that I took my blinders off for the first time in a year and looked at anything but my transplant patient.

What I focused on first was April at the Cape. Although it's still cold, raw, and rainy in Maine, April isn't "the cruellest month" at all to me. The crocuses are mostly up, daffodil shoots are beginning to emerge between the last patches of snow, and the bulk of the woolens are back in the attic. I was delighted to be back for at least the last week of it, and even though I should have been worrying about getting moved to the cottage for Sam, I couldn't bring myself to. I endlessly shuffled the furniture around the new living room instead and, when I wasn't doing that, prevailed upon Malcolm's and Ruthie's already overtaxed sympathies to come for dinner so I could hold Gus. I think it was really Malcolm who opened my eyes to the narrowness of my character.

Ruthie had gone upstairs to Al's room to see her California treasures, Parker hadn't yet gotten home from the office, and Malcolm was sitting in a rocking chair rocking Gus.

Unlike Pokie, Malcolm has always had a fondness for babies, and despite his mustache and his pipe he was looking down at Gussie with exactly the same expression he'd had when he was six and I'd put Sam in his arms for the first time. Remembering that moment reduced me to the maudlin and entirely interrupted my table-setting.

"Oh, Malc, do you remember what you said when we brought Sam home after he was born?" I said, pausing by his chair with my table mats and silver. "You look just the way you did when you called him 'our everlasting Christmas present.'"

Malcolm has a strict conscience, and he looked up from Gus and said almost wistfully, "I guess so, Ma. I know that's what I kept saying he had to go on being all this winter. I only wish Ruthie and I had been able to help more."

That sentence brought such a flood of memories of what he and Ruthie and everyone had done that I couldn't say anything. I thought of Ruthie, eight months along, trudging out into the snow and the cold to take Al to school, and of the letters she'd written, before she and Malcolm moved, that started: "Malcolm is out shoveling snow, but Al and I are cuddled up in her bed." I thought of Tina saying over the phone, "I've got the best brothers in all the world," and I thought of Pokie using the money he was saving for a car to come to California to see Sam. I thought of Al saying "See ya, Mum" as casually as if I were going away for the night, when I was actually leaving for three weeks; and I thought of the letter Charlie had written Sam before he got his heart: "Our new room at the Cape is okay, but I haven't got anybody to sing 'Wild Weed Flower' with, so it was pretty dull over Christmas. Get yourself fixed up and GET HOME. You are the greatest, Joe!"

And finally I thought of what Al had told me coming home on the plane. I'd gotten nervous as we got close to Portland.

"Al," I'd said, "how the hell am I going to tell Daddy and Dottie about moving to the cottage? Everybody's going to think we're crazy, moving five hundred feet down the field for the summer"; and she'd said, "Oh, everybody knew we would. Dottie bought Charlie some paint, and he painted dining room furniture down there the whole week he was home for vacation."

All the things that everybody had done were right there in front of me. "Oh, Malcolm, don't," I cried. "Don't ever say that. Everybody had to help, and the magic of it all is that everybody did," and suddenly, and for the first time, I really understood Lois Christopherson's third criterion for having a heart transplant.

It had sounded almost clinical when she said it: "A recipient has to be a good risk physically in the first place, psychologically sound in the second, and, third, has to have strong family support throughout."

Right then, talking to Malcolm in the kitchen, I knew that without all of us, however much Sam had wanted to live, he couldn't have. If I'd been worried about Alix, he would have known and felt he was hurting her. Thanks to everyone at home, I hadn't had to. Thanks to Unkie, Parker had been able to leave his business, and Sam had never had to worry that his father was upset about that.

And it wasn't just all of us at home. Aunt Roz, Uncle Bill, Dottie, Sam's friends, and our friends, everyone who'd kept things going at the house when we couldn't ourselves, Kent, Stanford, the nurses, even people who only knew of Sam by hearsay — the "thanks to" list went on and on, and, hurtling it out at Malcolm, I realized I'd never actually said thank you to anyone. Although no one had ever made me feel I should, I had to begin.

"Oh, thank you, Gussie, for being born and making us all feel good," I cried, swooping him out of his father's arms.

When I went to a Kent trustees' meeting and the rector emeritus opened it with a prayer for Sam, I realized, with a lump in my throat, that I hadn't even properly thanked God.

I felt very humble that time at home, and the only soul I didn't feel grateful to was Moriah. Admittedly she had helped the summer Sam was sick by walking with me and listening to me, but for that I had already thanked her, and she had now abandoned deerslaying for porcupine-pouncing and was my despair.

Rozzie and I had taken a walk with the dogs at her house one day, and when a car drove into the yard I knew it was Pokie, because he exclaimed in horrified tones, "Mother, what are you *doing*?"

I couldn't see his expression, because I was sitting on

Moriah's rear, hunched over Rozzie, who was sitting on her shoulders. On top of Rozzie too, but at Moriah's head, looking toward her tail, was Uncle Billy, pulling out porcupine quills with his pliers. Only when the last of thirty-two were removed did we stand up to see Parker III in his state of shock.

"My God, Uncle Bill," he said with relief. "I didn't see the dog. It looked as if you and Mother were beating up Aunt Roz. I thought it was some kinky 'in' thing she'd brought back from California."

Oh, I didn't want to go back there. The apple blossoms were bursting into the windows of our new bedroom the day I had to leave, it was 70 degrees, and, from what Tina had reported of Sam when she came home, a mother was the last thing Sam needed — or wanted.

She and Sam had had a ball with the nurses. He'd bought himself a bright yellow madras suit at Brooks Brothers in San Francisco, had beaten her 9–7 their last set of tennis, and, according to Unkie, the next Oak Creek visitor, was becoming a bon vivant.

Parker had relieved Tina of her duties with Sam, and Unkie had dropped by the currently bachelor pad at Oak Creek for a few days. He called me up when he got home.

"Parker thinks Sam's restless," he said. "Seven sets of tennis a day, hobnobbing with Jim Plunkett and the Forty-Niners, and almost wearing me out doing San Francisco aren't enough. He's taking him to Lake Tahoe to gamble."

I was out when Sam and Parker called the next day. "It wasn't even collect," Dottie told me. "They say they're winning and very rich."

Twenty-four hours later Parker called again. He did not sound prosperous at all.

"Are you still alive? Did Sam get any sleep?" I asked nervously — and with good reason, for the sight of a green baize tabletop obliterates time from Parker's mind.

"Just barely and not much," he croaked. "We got caught in a blizzard in the Sierra and had to buy chains for the car, but what a blast. Old Heart Transplant One-twenty can handle himself anywhere. I just wish you could have seen him plunking down the bets."

"I'm glad I didn't," I said sourly. "You're a hell of a nurse," and all the way to San Francisco I suspected I was going to be a terrible comedown from Tina and Unkie and Parker.

I also suspected that heart transplanting had left its mark on Parker's formerly paternal relationship with his fifth child. The trip to Lake Tahoe sounded more like the jolly boys off on a spree than a proper father-son expedition.

When I got to Oak Creek I discovered that Parker was a hell of a housekeeper, too. It wasn't that things weren't clean, but the formerly well-filled cupboards were empty. Every glass, plate, pot, pan, and utensil was strewn over the kitchen counters.

"It's called the energy game, Mum," Sam said, as if that explained everything, and when I asked disagreeably what energy total chaos was saving, he and his father said "Ours" with such complacence that I knew they too suspected I was going to be a terrible comedown. "Comrades" best described Sam and Parker as they walked off together to the pool to escape my displeasure, and, grumpy as I was, I couldn't help wondering how Sam had brought about Parker's lack of paternalism.

I found out that night when Parker and I were talking. Sam had set his father straight the very first day they shared living quarters at Oak Creek, as he had me.

343

"Have you taken your medicines?" Parker had asked him, as they started down toward the tennis courts for their first game.

Sam had whirled on him. "Don't you ever ask me if I've taken my medicines again," he had said fiercely. "It's my body; I'll worry about it."

And Parker said to me, "I never will again, you know."

The night we moved into the plastic, Parker had put the return halves of the three undated, first-class, round-trip tickets into an envelope. "We won't use these till we take Sammy home," he'd said, and once in January I'd looked in the envelope and felt such despair that I'd never touched it again. When I got back to California, the tickets were dated, and the date was June 3.

"Don't get excited," Parker cautioned when he showed them to me. "The hospital only said sometime the first part of June, but our lease runs out on the first, and I just picked the third as a good day because it's the anniversary of everything — six months to the day from when Sam got accepted."

The hospital didn't seem to get carried away by sentiment. After Parker left, the clinic days dragged by without anything more than a "We'll see" or a "Maybe."

"Hell," Sam complained drearily after one trip to clinic, "Randy was supposed to go home the twenty-fifth, and he's still here," and he appropriated the living-room sofa with all the lethargy of pretransplant time at the plastic.

Parker and I have a friend who, when asked where he was during the Second War, says, "Guadalcanal for three years, five months, fifteen days, eleven hours, seven minutes, and two-and-a-half seconds." That's what it was like at Oak Creek that last time.

Sam looked marvelous. He weighed 150 pounds, each one approved by the hospital as muscle, not fluid. Between sofa sessions he exercised religiously to keep himself that way, but I knew that all he was thinking about was going home.

It was the same for me. The final biopsy he had to have hadn't even been scheduled by May 29, the day Charlie graduated from Trinity without us. The weather had been horrible, and although I'd written optimistically in my diary on the twenty-eighth, "Could it possibly be only 1, 2, 3, 4, 5 more days in beautiful downtown Palo Alto?" on the twenty-ninth I wrote, "I doubt it!"

It was a Sunday, and Sam was beset by gloom because June 2, the day that would have been his Kent graduation, was fast approaching. All his friends had called to know if there was a chance of his making it.

"Have one for me after you get your diplomas, you guys," he said as he hung up, and, slouching back to the sofa: "Oh, God, I wish I could be there to see those guys finish up. They'll all be gone next year when I go back."

It was almost the last straw when everybody called us from Trinity after the graduation. All I could think after we hung up was, We've got to get home — we've got to get back together again soon or everything's going to fall apart; and when Sam sullenly declined to play tennis with me, I stamped off for a long walk. Two large blisters later I came back, and for the first time since the night before he got his heart I let him have it.

"You are rude," I said. "Rude, rude, rude! It's hard enough being away from home without you being so damned ugly," and I watched the tears that sprang to his eyes without a twinge until he said, "Oh, Mum, I want to go home," and I started to cry too.

Parker came out on the thirty-first. "All three of us got here together, and that's how we're going home," he'd said, but we had no idea when we could leave, although Sam did have his biopsy that day.

We gave a farewell party for all the nurses we'd met and their Hims the next night and not surprisingly, while the party lasted, not knowing when or if we'd be leaving didn't bother any of us. Sam reigned supreme in his kingdom; the rest of us sat around on chairs or on the floor and enjoyed watching him.

"Well, now that you all know my mother can't cook," he said cheerfully, after the remains of dinner had been deposited in the kitchen, "I have a few thank-yous to make to the best nurses in the whole world. At this rate I may still be here for another six months, but right now, tonight, remembering what I looked like when you started with me, and" — flexing his arms — "looking at me now, you gotta admit you did a good job."

He toasted each one in turn and finally pulled out from beneath the chair where he'd been sitting a huge paper bag.

"This," he announced, "is for Lynn, because she signed up for me before she even knew how great I was. It's a wedding present," and out of the bag came his hooked rug.

The huge lion was still lacking ears, and the background which was to have been azure blue was not. "Here," Sam said, handing it to Lynn, "you can finish it yourself. Rug hooking's not my thing."

Lynn threw her arms around him and kissed him, and even though he bent down to hug her, she had to stand on tiptoe to reach him. She was laughing and crying all at once. "Oh, Sam," she said, "what are we ever going to do without you? You're so awful!"

The next day I cleaned the apartment and tried to pack. We'd been given grace to stay in it till the second, but that was it, and we still didn't know if we could go home. It was the plastic all over again, only worse. We could hardly go home on the plane with the orange dishpan packed with our belongings, and when Sam came back from clinic with two huge, bulging paper bags, I felt defeated.

"My God," I said, "I thought they were going to mail you the six-month supply of medicines," as he spread out on the table nineteen large glass bottles, twenty-two small ones, and six cardboard boxes of potassium packets.

"They're going to," he said. "This is just to keep me going till I get to Maine," and he went off to the pool for a swim.

Judy came and added a book to the pile and Kathy a foot-tall jade plant.

"You don't have to take it home, but God would be cross," she said. The jade, it seemed, was very metaphysical. She'd dropped its pot in March, when she heard the news that Sam might have to have another heart, and, as she scooped up the dirt and the broken pieces and the plant, she and God had come to an understanding. If the jade plant lived, so would Sam. The light in her apartment was lousy for jades. It would be safer with me.

"What's that?" Parker demanded, looking at the plant.

"That's Sam," I said. "Don't touch it."

"Is it going home?" he asked with obvious dismay, and without a moment's hesitation and with one voice, Judy, Kathy, and I said "Yes!"

Sometime during that day which seemed to have no possible end, the lady who ran the Oak Creek health club called and told Sam the tennis pro wanted him down at the courts, and just after he left the phone rang again.

"This is Joan from the clinic," a voice said. "May I speak to Sam?"

Feeling like the spider talking to the fly, I asked if I could take a message. The fly was too sophisticated.

"No," Joan said firmly. "The message is for Sam."

It was almost three o'clock when Sam returned with an embarrassed grin and a large brown canvas tennis bag. "Gawd," he said, "they didn't have to do that." A card attached to the bag wished him the very best of luck from the tennis pro and the lady at the health club and included an invitation to stay with them if he ever needed a bed in California.

I was so overcome I almost forgot for a second to tell him to call the clinic, and once I did, and he had, I fell apart. I forget what happened next, but I know that at five o'clock, with the new brown bag bursting with Sam's medicines, and with the jade plant tucked in my arms, we turned in our keys and left Oak Creek forever.

"Going home, going home," I sang, to Sam and Parker's dismay, all the way to the airport and all that night at the airport motel. I was still singing it intermittently the next morning as we approached TWA's X-ray machines to have our carry-on bags examined.

As Sam strode ahead of us, the brown bag slung over his shoulder, his pack on his back, I grabbed Parker's arm and said, "Just look at him!" It didn't seem possible that he was the boy we'd pushed through the same terminal six months before, slumped in a wheelchair, the huge envelope of X-rays in his lap. Chipmunk cheeks under a California tan and a golden beard *were* beautiful. Everybody said that now that the massive doses of prednisone he'd taken during rejection were being tapered down, his cheeks would go down too, but I didn't care; I'd had enough tortured-saint looks to last me a lifetime. Dottie herself couldn't have found flaws. He looked, thanks to Stanford and Dr. Shumway, as if he'd never been sick a day in his life.

The woman at the TWA X-ray machine must have thought so too. After the brown bag went through, she seized it before we could say a word.

"It's packed too closely to see what's in it," she said. "I'll have to open it," and she did. "What are these?" she demanded. It was clear that she thought she'd nailed a pusher.

Parker rushed forward to explain, but Sam was way ahead of him.

"I'm a heart transplant and those are my medicines," he said, and he pulled out his medical card and showed her his wrist bracelet. "If you have any questions, you can call this number at Stanford Medical Center, but don't touch those pills. I need them."

After several close scrutinies of the card and the bracelet by an additional security guard, we passed through. "Well, once a heart transplant, always a heart transplant, I guess," Sam said jauntily, but the whole thing was still upsetting me when we got to the gate.

He was different, he was always going to be different, but suddenly, as I looked up to see all his nurses rushing toward us, I wasn't upset anymore. With Sam in charge it was going to be a difference that would be easy for everybody to live with. His nurses loved him as we did — and as his friends at home would — because he was, heart transplant, medicines, side effects, and all, Sam.

I looked at the almond-shaped eyes filled with little tears, and the dark ones that crinkled at the corners, and the violet ones, and saying good-bye to them was saying good-bye to the children at Christmastime all over again. I couldn't do it, and I was still gulping back the tears as our plane took off.

The kind of mind that likes washing woodwork and reads the ends of books first is not well adapted to great triumph. Was triumph laughing our heads off and toasting each other with champagne in the first-class cabin, or was it explaining to the stewardess why we were? Perhaps triumph was the huge bottle of wine, wrapped in a TWA napkin, that she presented to Sam as we left the plane in Boston, and the silver pens that the businessmen, sitting in front of him, insisted that he accept with their compliments.

Triumph, I knew, was when Sam walked through Gate Two of Portland's International Jetport, to be smothered in hugs by Aunt Roz and Uncle Bill, Ruthie, Malcolm, Pokie, Charlie, Tina, Alix, Unkie, and Dana.

His beard bristling like Grizzly Adams's, Heart Transplant 120 held out his arms to receive little Malcolm Augustus. While his words may have lacked the splendor of a conquering hero's, they were none the less memorable.

"Hi there, baby," said Uncle Sam, popping his eyes at it. "Boogie, boogie, boogie!"

I know too that triumph was the picture that Parker took that night at the coming-home party Dottie and the children had organized. The dogs refused to stop tearing around; but lined up in the new living room that Sam had never seen were Malcolm with an arm around Pokie who had an arm around Tina who had an arm around Charlie who had an arm around Sam. The transplant himself had pulled a grinning Alix squarely in front of him, and his left arm was crooked around her neck. Underneath Pokie's and Tina's arms crouched Ruthie, holding Gus.

I looked at them all standing there, and, even though

Sam didn't have a dragon's tail draped over his shoulder or a two-headed bulldog obediently at heel, I knew he was at the very top of the glass mountain. There seemed to be all kinds of room up there for the rest of us too, and, if no one had spotted the princess yet, she would surely turn up sooner or later.

The next morning Parker and I waved good-bye to Sam as he set forth in the old blue Volvo for a Kent graduation party. The last time he had driven off in that direction he had been dying, and, although the Volvo looked as sick and tired as ever, a gloriously sturdy brown arm waved back at us.

"Thursday's child has far to go," I said, squeezing Parker's hand, but he didn't seem to hear.

"Full circle," he said, as the car disappeared out of sight beyond the pond. "By God, we've come full circle."

Epilogue
The "one last summer" that Sam requested the year he got his heart is rapidly turning into a third. Our new house glistens with fresh paint on the outside and with polish on the inside, and yet I leave it each May, like some demented migratory bird, to arrive at the cottage armed with pails and mops and cleaning supplies. Moving five hundred feet involves as much labor as moving ten miles away, and from time to time the folly of it all sinks in, and I rebel.

Traditionally, Rozzie and I start to open our summer dwellings on a Sunday, so that the weekly family picnic breaks up the horrid discoveries of a winter's absence. That picnic always takes place on the sea side of the cottage, on the lawn on top of the cesspool. This year it didn't, and it was I who shattered the custom. It wasn't just that the dead stalks of last year's marigolds were depressing. It wasn't even that there really wasn't any lawn to picnic on. (Although most of the winter's accumulation of sand and rocks and plastic bottles have been raked away by May, the chief ground cover at the cottage consists of flakes of white paint — sandblasted off the clapboards by storms — until the grass finally gets courageous enough to poke its way up late in June.) The fact that the cottage's gas heater had refused to ignite — forcing me to slosh all morning through pools of water from leaking drains in 40-degree temperatures — wasn't what caused my revolt; nor was it the heavy mist that had enveloped us for days.

It was the tail of the dead mouse I had found on the attic stairs. When I picked it up, it detached itself from its owner, and I ran shrieking up the path to Rozzie's.

"That does it," I said flatly when I found her in the kitchen. "I am never going near that place again. From now on I am going to live in my house like a civilized human being."

To placate me the Tea House, with its sheltering wall, was selected as our picnic site, and Aunt Roz, Uncle Bill, Charlie, Alix, Malcolm, Gussie, Parker and the dogs and I assembled there at noon. Ruthie had taken the new baby, Beth, to her tenth reunion at Milton, and Louise was missing: she had departed for the Wind Rivers of Wyoming to study the sixteen osprey nests there under a grant from Yale's Forestry School. We were also lacking Tina — now properly diplomaed and a travel agent for an international sports agency in Connecticut — and the heart transplant, who was still at college. Pokie and his Her were expected momentarily; Susan is an artist, working in, of all unlikely places, Kansas City, but Pokie, who had gone to Boston to meet her plane, had assured us that the picnic was on their schedule.

Still jaundiced by the dismemberment of the mouse, I found my resolve to abandon the annual summer upheaval was strengthened as I looked at Charlie, who until now had always been the mainstay of my move. Having almost sunk on a small coastal oil tanker in a terrible storm the winter after Sam came home, he has quit the sea for Connecticut's rivers and become the freshman crew coach at Trinity. My initial relief at such relatively safe employment was overcome by dismay as I realized that he wouldn't be around to help this year.

"I have to leave right after lunch," Charlie announced. "Crew practice at six."

Huddled next to the little airtight stove, I decided to make my pronouncement. "We are not moving to the cottage this summer. I am too old," I was just beginning in a firm and rational voice, when Alix, clutching two-year-old Gus to keep him from climbing out a window, cried, "Here they come!"

None of us had seen Susan since New Year's, and we had missed her. We are all as unsubtle as underwear buttons, and Susan, who is dark and beautiful, adds immeasurable mystery to our family gatherings. We underwear buttons rushed out cheering just as she and Pokie came through the little green door in the stone wall. It was a perfectly normal — if noisy — family welcoming, but two minutes later, when Pokie, calmly lounging against the fireplace, said, "I think you all might be interested to know that Susan and I are going to be married this fall," regulation pandemonium turned to bedlam.

Rozzie and I jumped up and down, hugging first one of them and then the other in such confusion that we ended up hugging each other; Alix, in imitation of Susan, tried to look mysterious but ended up giggling; Malcolm and Charlie beat Pokie on the back; and Parker, with proper Parkerish dignity, planted a gentlemanly kiss on Susan's cheek. The dogs started barking, and Uncle Bill had to roar, "Oh, God, Pokie, how can I fire you now, when you're saving for the ring?" in order to be heard at all. It must have been a good five minutes before anyone noticed Gussie, rolling around between the dogs on the old bed that serves as a couch and crowing, in language learned at Christmastime from his Uncle Sam, "Cool, man, cool."

By nightfall everyone in the family had heard the news. Ruthie, Louise, and Tina reacted with predictable and ecstatic hysteria, but Sam, though obviously pleased, sounded stunned.

"Pokie? Married? Ya gotta be kidding."

Only Dottie maintained her regal calm. "I've known for ages," she said when I called her at her house. "When a Poole buys four airline tickets in one year to go see someone, it's love."

There's nothing like romance to banish depressions. I had completely forgotten about my determination to live sensibly in one house, until Alix said, just as she was going up to bed, "Oh, Mummy, can't we move? It won't be right being up here in the summer."

I looked at her, surprised. The dear familiar roundness of Big Al, the consolation of Parker's and my declining years, has long since melted away. I'm almost getting used to this tall sultry brunette who has become the family fashion consultant, but, until she said that, I hadn't realized how much wiser than I she was getting to be. Only fourteen, but like Sam two years before, she knew that nothing that is loved ought to be abandoned just because it's the sensible thing to do.

I threw my arms around her, crying, "Of course we're moving!" And in my heart I knew that the cottage is where I always want to be in the summer, where everything is just the way it always has been. It's only seasonally and spasmodically that I forget. Charlie's crew season is almost over, and he and Sam will both be home in less than a month. Tina and Louise will be back for vacations, and, with Ruthie and Malcolm, and Gussie and Beth, and Pokie, and now Susan, in and out, the cottage is where we belong, with the aunts and the dogs and the children running back and forth between houses and the pool in the middle. There's no better place in the world for keeping things the way they always have been.

I knew that as soon as we moved there after we got back from California two years ago. The upstairs bathtub was leaking just as it has always leaked, and, avoiding the familiar puddle it leaves on the kitchen floor just as he always has, Sam appeared at seven o'clock the next morning, unkempt and uncombed, in his boxcar-unloading clothes. One bowl of cornflakes and a grunted "See ya" later, he had departed for the W. H. Shurtleff Company. It was as if we'd never been away, and as if the whole awful summer before had never happened.

I don't mean for a minute that we ever forgot that we had a genuine, certified, braceleted heart transplant living with us. We couldn't because, if Sam had devoted the first four months of his new life to getting well and strong, he spent the second four setting historic and often nerve-racking precedents. While we don't know that he was the first heart transplant to unload boxcars, we suspect that he was the first to water ski, and he was, we're sure — and with his mother in a state of collapse — the first to jump twenty feet into the ocean from the roof of a tugboat's pilothouse. As his nurse Judy told him just after he got out of the hospital, "There are a lot of things you may be able to do that you thought you couldn't, Sam." Going into the ocean without getting an infection was one of them. Having girls in his room at Kent was not.

356

He is undoubtedly the first transplant to be put on probation at boarding school for that error in judgment. "Why didn't you tell them to get out?" I said indignantly, when the news broke that three girls — not for love, but to escape the night watchmen — had burst into the room shared by Sam and two other boys at one o'clock in the morning, shortly after school started.

"Christ, Mum, you wouldn'ta wanted them to think I was a queer or something, would you?" he replied.

Kent was very good to Sam. Not only did it let him keep his beard, but Hart Perry let him have a car because he had to visit a cardiologist in the next town twice a week. In Sam's opinion, Parker was not at all good to him. When the old blue Volvo died of its infirmities, Parker replaced it with ("Oh, gross, Dad!") an ancient gold Dodge Polara, which caught on fire just before Thanksgiving, en route to a doctor's appointment. The cardiologist, passing by in his own car, saw Sam's in flames at a gas station and rushed to the rescue.

"Sam," he said, wearily mopping his brow when the fire was out, "tell your father to get you a safe car before I need a heart transplant myself."

"A sports car would be nice, Dad," Sam said when he phoned that night.

"The Dodge is still running, isn't it?" Parker replied. "What the hell are you complaining about? Now, when I was your age . . ."

It was scarcely a month later that a young master at Kent who had taken a shine to Tina borrowed the car to drive to Trinity to take her out for dinner. On the way home, he demolished not only a deer but a good part of the front of the golden Dodge.

Poole cars, including mine, never cost more than four

hundred dollars, and no one was surprised to hear, after Sam clanked his way home for Christmas vacation, that it would cost more to repair his than to replace it. Well adjusted to Parker's automotive philosophy, "You learn a lot about cars when they break down," he was understandably less than overjoyed a few days later to hear that his father had found a substitute.

"Whatta ya bet, a 1965 Valiant?" he sighed, as he departed with Freddie Gemmer for the appointed used-car lot.

An hour later there was wild tooting outside the kitchen and the roar of an engine that sounded like no Poole car I had ever heard. Dottie and I rushed to the door to see Sam leaping out of a little green machine, his cool for once abandoned.

"Dad's flipped out," he was shrieking. "My God, he's flipped! It's a Porsche — a 1974 nine-fourteen Porsche. I don't believe it — he's gotta have flipped!"

Parker looked very sheepish when he came home. "I don't care," he said, before I could even begin to tease him. "I got a good deal on it, and what the hell? If you could have seen the look on Sam's face when he saw it."

I did see the look on Sam's face when he graduated from Kent, and I heard the cheers of the student body when he passed through its ranks. Despite the fact that a rejection in April had put him back on massive doses of prednisone and his cheeks were quite round, he had shaved off his beard. ("Who the hell wants to stick out like a sore thumb?" he had explained to his startled relations at the family party the night before.) Dressed, along with the rest of the sixth form, in a blue blazer and remarkably clean white pants, his blond hair a split-fraction of an inch above his collar (just enough to spare him a haircut), he was as anonymous as anyone in a state of ecstasy can be. His Adidas were even tied. The moment he'd yearned for for so long, lying huddled on the sofa in the plastic apartment, had finally come. Remembering all the times I'd thought it never could, and sitting amid faculty members, deans, and even the headmaster — with the black serge and velvet-hooded dignities of Trusteeship upon my shoulders — I disgraced myself and cried.

Already in the back of our car ("You wouldn't want me to crud up mine, Dad!") were his belongings, and mixed in with the books and the laundry and the stereo were the tangible triumphs of the year. There was a new varsity letter. It wasn't for rowing; his ankles had given out in training. It certainly wasn't for football or hockey, which were strictly against transplant rules. It was for swimming and for giving the team, the citation said, "heart." There was a copy of the *Kent News,* which described Sam's performance in a melodrama in the role of "the villain with absolutely no heart at all" as "experienced," and there were two letters of acceptance from colleges. I'd cried over those triumphs too, but they couldn't touch the look on Sam's face when he graduated.

The college acceptances had come in April. One was from Trinity; not in vain had we called her "bless-ed" all these years. The other, unbelievably, was from Stanford. There had never been any question in our minds that Stanford University Medical Center had heart, but it had seemed wishful thinking to expect that Stanford University would too. It might be argued that the admissions department simply got worn down by the barrage of letters and calls on Sam's behalf. It has even been rudely suggested that his SAT and achievement test scores got lost, but I prefer to think that Sam got accepted because Stanford had heart.

With the Medical Center just a three-minute bike ride away, it was where he belonged.

On Saturday at eight o'clock in the morning, September 9, 1978, the little green Porsche was packed to the gunwales. Having accomplished the packing after being nagged by his father for a full month to get organized, Sam was thrilled with himself. Planting a kiss on my cheek, he swung out of the kitchen door at the cottage to start his drive to California. He was to meet up with two other carloads of Stanford-bound Kent students in Connecticut.

"See ya, Dad," he said and, having grasped his pajama-clad father's hand, started the engine.

Parker walked around the car, making one last check of its condition. His eye caught the license plate. "Sam," he roared, "You're not going anywhere. You didn't get the damned car registered!"

The heroine of the day was the clerk of the Town of Cape Elizabeth, who abandoned a Saturday shopping trip to open the town safe and reregister the heart transplant. It took some time to find her.

"See ya, Mum. See ya, Dad," Sam said five hours later, as cheerfully as though nothing had happened, and drove away.

So life with Sam for the most part hasn't been any different from life with any nineteen- or twenty-year-old. His bathroom looks as if it had just been hit by the fuzz in a drug raid. In his bedroom, it is hard to locate his bed. When he's home I tell him daily that I am going to have a bumper sticker made saying HEART TRANSPLANTS ARE SLOBS; and it doesn't distress him at all. Very little seems to.

"Hi, there, fat face," said a girl he hadn't seen since he'd gotten his heart, as he walked by her table in a bar, just after he got home to Maine.

"I'm sorry to hear that you have a social disease," he responded, bowing courteously to her and passing on.

Even the things that go badly for him rarely get him down. Not once have I heard him bemoan his diet, which away from home seems to consist chiefly of salads. Standard boarding-school fare was out of the question for him at Kent last year, and he cooked for himself in the kitchen at the school infirmary. At Stanford there's no problem. "Everyone out there's into all this health food junk anyway," he says. Equally, I have never heard him protest the things he has to do to keep himself going. I found a huge old leather shoe satchel of Mother's to hold his medicines, and he slings it into his car, when he sets off on a trip, just as casually as he tosses in his sleeping bag. But if his medicines are what keep him alive, they are also the source of most of his miseries. The things he can do but thought he couldn't are balanced, courtesy of the medicines, by the ones he can't do but thought he could. Long before he got his heart, he had accepted the automatic ban on contact sports, but he had no idea how many other restrictions would creep up on him. The strange thing is that, while the medicines taken by different heart transplants are virtually the same, they seem to affect each one differently. Randy's complaints, his mother and I agree, are not Sam's. Sam's problem has been — and is — bruising, bleeding, and bad bones.

"Had twenty stitches in my left leg today. Fell off my bike. Some dumb girl ran into me," he is apt to announce casually over the phone one night.

And two days later, "Christ, I climbed on a table at the Beta House last night and cut the other leg." Eighteen more to repair that injury.

As a rough estimate, I'd say close to three hundred

stitches have gone into those long bony legs in the course of the past two years. They add up fast when fifty go in at once, as they did last week. The doctors who know him sew him up with resignation ("Not again, Sam!"), but there have been others — in Farmington, Maine, and on Nantucket Island, for example — who have approached the task tremulously. ("Never sewn up a heart transplant before," they mutter, stitching away, between mounds of scar tissue and bulging purple hematomas, at the paper-thin skin.)

Although he never talks about it, I know it was a blow for Sam when his ankles went. Thanks to prednisone, the damaged joints of heart transplants are damaged for good, and Sam has given up running, rowing, and tennis for the most part. Although he still skis a little, ski boots, he says, are not designed for heart transplants, and he had to switch last summer from boxcar unloading to the machine shop of the W. H. Shurtleff Company. He is the gofer.

"Gopher?" I asked when I heard his new title. "Yeah, I go fer this and I go fer that," and while gofering is easier on his ankles, it's always plain that, when he's on his feet, Sam hurts. There is one notable exception. When the music starts, Sam dances. The beat or the girl or both must provide temporary anesthesia.

The rejection he had the April before he graduated was his third. He had his second, complicated by a lung infection, the August after he came home. Both were successfully treated by Dr. Wakely in Maine, acting along with telephoned advice from Stanford, but, though I never forget for one second that Sam is a miracle, those setbacks were even harsher reminders than bruises and crumbling bones and cuts that a heart transplant is not a cure.

I think the third rejection was the cruelest for him. He came home from a spring vacation cruise on a friend's boat in the Bahamas, and it was plain that the world was his oyster. He couldn't wait for spring term. He'd taken his last exams, he'd been accepted at college, and he was as well-muscled, tanned, and flat of cheek as any self-respecting heart transplant should have a right to be. A week later his voltage plunged. He drove home from Kent that afternoon and flew to California two hours later to have a biopsy, as Stanford requested. The biopsy was clear, and, still on the crest of the wave and only twenty-five milligrams of prednisone, he drove back to Kent, one hour after his plane landed in Portland.

Two weeks later he was back in Maine. There was no question this time that he was rejecting, and his prednisone was increased to one hundred milligrams. When he got home from Dr. Wakely's office, he put his head down on the kitchen table and wept.

"Oh, Mum, why?" he sobbed. "When I just get things going right, why does everything have to go wrong?"

But he knows why, just as all the rest of us do. The odd thing is that Kathy's secret pact with God, the jade plant, seems to understand too. Both times that Sam rejected, I watched, horrified and disbelieving, as its leaves began to shrivel and turn yellow. When he stopped rejecting, it stopped dying, and, while I know it's absurd to run howling with joy to the telephone to tell everyone that the jade plant has a blossom or that it has put out a new shoot, I can't help doing it. It is Sam's weathervane, and, as long as its leaves are green and glossy, the future doesn't seem to be all that formidable. I know that there is the possibility of an operation to fuse his ankles in the future and another, somewhere down the line, to remove the cataracts that are beginning to form in his eyes. There is always talk of skin grafts for his legs. Someone asked Rozzie once, "How can he bear it?" and she answered, just as Sam or any of us would, "When you consider the alternative, it's very bearable."

My ghosts know that. Whenever I start to get upset about Sam, they flock to remind me how lucky he is. The boy who gave him his heart is always there, and Rick Taylor, the backup recipient, who died waiting for his heart to come along. There is Burpee, and Mr. Terrence, and poor Jeff Ogilvey, the man who was afraid to have a transplant. (Even a second heart, put in just after Sam came home to Maine, failed him, and he died.)

The ghosts are in my mind a lot, and, in the middle of the night when Sam is away, there is the dread but certain knowledge that no heart transplant has ever lived for more than ten years. I lie awake and worry until I begin to think that, short of his bad ankles and his cuts, Stanford says Sam is just as healthy as he was two years ago. I hear him saying, "I'm gonna keep going and going, and I'm gonna outlive them all," and I know he will, and I go back to sleep.

When he's home I haven't got time to worry about him. Just listening to him carry on is a full-time occupation: witness our trip on Parker's tug, the M.V. *Victoria*, to visit Tina at the little island where she was working last summer.

"Can I have a few friends on board when you come down to Squirrel, Dad?" Tina had asked her father earlier in the summer.

"Of course," Parker had responded. "That's why we're coming," but the captain and the eleven family members who made up his crew had difficulty classifying the seventy-four people who swarmed on board for an all-day picnic as "a few friends." Only Sam remained unrattled enough to enjoy the situation properly.

Feeling much less adequate than Our Lord with his loaves and fishes, Rozzie and I were worming our way toward the multitudes on the stern with plates of cookies when we spotted Sam in the center of a huge group of little boys.

"How did you get all those scars all over you?" one little boy was asking, looking nervously up at Sam's chest and down at his legs.

Sam rolled his eyes. "Sharks," he said, and his voice was ominous. "It was sharks. Right here at Squirrel Island. I hadn't swum ten feet away from the boat this morning when they were after me. If you guys go swimming, be sure you take a needle and thread along. I'da bled to death if I hadn't sewed myself right up."

All Sam's audience had swum out to the boat. Tina had to row it ashore in its entirety. "Damn you, Sam," she said, as she set forth with the fourth load of juveniles.

I am well adjusted to that Sam, and I'm even learning to adjust to the new California Sam who is bronzed twelve months of the year. Parker and I went out twice to visit him this year. Both times we partied with his nurses — who scold him when he cuts himself and pat him nervously when he looks too thin — and with his new friends from college.

"I know Sam's friends worry more about him than he does about himself," the mother of one of them told me this spring when we were in Palo Alto. "They just can't understand how he can be so happy about everything."

I didn't know her well enough to tell her that I had finally learned how he could. In the fall when we'd visited him, we had dinner with a boy who had complained sadly that it had just been discovered that his girl had diabetes.

"She's really shook up," he said. "It's awful to think of having to put up with insulin for the rest of your life."

Sam looked at him for a minute and then he said, "Hell, what's she got to complain about? She's alive, isn't she? She oughta realize that something that seems like the end of the world can be the best thing that ever happened to you. It was for me."

At Stanford, Sam has taken to the stage and was even given an opportunity to work in professional theater for the summer. He says he decided to come home instead because he misses us, but I suspect that his nine-month accumulation of dirty laundry was a factor. I'm thrilled with Sam the actor, though I doubt I will ever grow accustomed to Sam the scholar. "A, A-minus, A-minus, B-plus, and Pass on a pass-fail course," he announced jubilantly over the phone this spring, after Parker and I had said yes, of course we wanted to hear his semester grades.

"I think he's had a brain transplant," I said nervously after we hung up.

A lot of things Sam does, though, aren't what anybody ever had in mind. I'm sure that when Dr. Shumway started his research, he never expected to have a heart transplant write a letter like the one Sam wrote Tina just before spring vacation this year. "Dear Tina," it said. "I'm goin' down to Mehico to be a beach surfin' Daddy-o-o!!! I'm gonna catch the curl, shoot the tube, and ride the wave — that's beach surfin', Daddy-o talk. Ten of us going — oughta be a good time as long as they don't throw us in jail. . . ."

They didn't, and I can't wait for the "beach surfin' Daddy-o" to get home. I can't even wait to get moved to the cottage, or for Fourth of July on the tugboat, or for this summer's Tea House dance. Pokie wants Uncle Bill's band to play, and Uncle Bill says he wants to sign up the topless girls from The Golden Banana, which he can't because Aunt Roz and Uncle Parker and I won't let him. Everyone will be home, all the Hims and Hers will be visiting, we'll all be busy watching Gussie learn to swim, and then, before we know it, there's Pokie's wedding. Short of the fact that the tailless mouse is right where I left him last Sunday, there's absolutely nothing to complain about.

Author's Note

Although I have changed the names of three of the transplant patients, the doctors in Portland, and the doctor at Massachusetts General Hospital who reviewed Sam's case, everyone else in the book retains his or her real name. It could never have been written without the aid of the following hordes of people, divided here into categories for simplicity's sake (many categories overlap).

As far as actually writing the book is concerned, my humblest thanks go to: Josephine Detmer, who found me an editor before I knew I had a story; to that editor, Genevieve Young, who could teach any idiot how to write a book; to Janet Baker, whose copyediting saved me from myself; to Michael Brandon, who gave me what my childhood teachers never could — an appreciation of grammar; and to my brother-in-law, William Richardson, who gave up a year's worth of Saturdays to pre-edit every chapter. Many of Sam's words are taken from tapes he made, and my undying gratitude goes to Alice Mary Pierce, who typed transcripts for me. (It was not an easy job. Sam did them in his car, which had engine trouble, in hopes that his father would hear the sinister noises and buy him a new one, and every word he said was muffled by bangs, thumps, and explosions.) I also thank her and my sister, Rosamond Richardson, for the hours of reading they did and the comments they made throughout the writing of the book. There would certainly never have been a book without Mabel Kinney, who did its typing, and her husband, Henry, who did her proofreading. The photographs are courtesy of a mélange of friends and family photographers: Ruth Poole and William Richardson, photographers-in-chief. The fact that there are photographs in the book at all is due chiefly to David Pratt, who was able to transpose a most eclectic gathering of colored snapshots into fine black-and-white prints.

The story's happy ending is due to so many people that it would take another book to list them all. In my east-of-the-Mississippi category are the doctors in Portland who took care of Sam before he went to California, their staffs who cheered him on, his doctors in Connecticut, and a special doctor, my cousin H. William Scott, Jr. Without his help Sam might never have gotten to Stanford in time. Our friends, our family, and Kent School, I know, are what got him from East to West and back again without once "losing heart." The Stanford list is just as long. The skill and the kindness of everybody there turned what started out as a nightmare into a wonderful part of our lives. I thank each and every one and only wish it were not too late to thank our first friend at the hospital, Sally Ricker, who died in 1978. She was a bright spot in a dreary two months.

For my part, I would never have a heart transplant without signing on Lynn Honma Iwane, Judith Lachenmeyer, Kathleen Rickert, Jessica Orfitelli, and David Bailey as my nurses and Tom Friedman as my EKG technician. I would certainly go only to Stanford, to be coped with by Dr. Norman Shumway, Dr. John Schroeder, and Dr. William Baumgartner and helped and cheered along by Lois Christopherson; I would insist that the Daileys and Randy return to Palo Alto to keep me company; and I would demand that the ICU staff be exactly the same as it was when Sam was there. I would hope that the cardiology clinic was still being superbly organized by Patricia Gamberg and Joan Miller. I would look forward to having it all arranged by Miss H. Knott.

And finally my thanks go to the hero of the book himself, Sam Poole, and to another hero, Parker Poole, Jr., my husband. They have been a part of every category.